A HANDBOO

PAEDIATRIC RAD

A HANDBOOK OF
PAEDIATRIC RADIOGRAPHY

CATHERINE GYLL, DSR

Westminster Children's Hospital and
Royal Alexandra Hospital
for Sick Children, Brighton

Illustrations by
SUSAN CLEAVER, DSR (R)

Westminster Children's Hospital

BLACKWELL SCIENTIFIC PUBLICATIONS
Oxford · London · Edinburgh · Melbourne

First published 1977

Gyll, Catherine
A handbook of paediatric radiography.
Bibl. – Index.
ISBN 0-632-00489-4
618.9'2007'572   RJ51.R3
Diagnosis, Radioscopic
Children – Diseases – Diagnosis

Distributed in the United States of America by
J.B. Lippincott Company, Philadelphia,
and in Canada by
J.B. Lippincott Company of Canada Ltd, Toronto.

Printed and bound in Great Britain by
Billing & Sons Limited,
Guildford, London and Worcester

CONTENTS

PREFACE

This book is not a complete textbook of paediatric radiography. It does not include those specialized radiological investigations for which a child is usually referred to a children's hospital. Its object is simply to make available to radiographers in general hospitals some ideas on how to achieve good radiographs at the first attempt.

All too often, babies and children are overexposed to radiation and other hazards, both emotional and physical, through repeated attempts to obtain acceptable radiographs, and a lack of basic knowledge of what is required. Radiographs of poor quality can be misleading, and cause mis-diagnosis.

It must always be remembered that to have to repeat a film because of lack of radiographic skill is to cause an extra dose of radiation to a young and growing human being.

My hope is that this book may be of help and guidance to young radiographers faced with their first paediatric patients.

Throughout the book I have used only the masculine personal pronouns for one very simple reason—it makes for easier reading.

I wish to thank my colleague Mrs Guelda Agyei for the idea of writing this book.

My thanks are due also to Dr Michael Fisher, radiologist, of the Royal Sussex County Hospital, and Dr Jane Fisher, anaesthetist, of the Royal Alexandra Hospital for Sick Children, for encouragement and many valuable suggestions in the initial stages.

I am greatly indebted to Dr Fritz Starer, radiologist, of the Westminster Children's Hospital, for reading and correcting many chapters; also to Mr Austin Brown, orthopaedic surgeon, Mr John Howat, paediatric surgeon, Mr Bernard Crymble, neuro-surgeon, and Mr Ian Crossman, orthodontist, all of the Royal Alexandra Hospital, Brighton; and Mr Brian Keane, physicist, of the Royal Sussex County Hospital, Brighton.

My radiographic colleagues in both hospitals made many helpful suggestions; the ward sisters and staff nurses provided me with much useful information.

Miss Marion Frank very kindly allowed me the use of the Middlesex Hospital School of Radiography post-graduate library, where much of the book was written.

Finally, I do not think it would ever have been finished without the generous help, encouragement and expert editorial advice of Miss Muriel Chesney.

CHAPTER I
X-RAYING CHILDREN

Children and infants differ as patients from adults in several ways, not just the obvious one of size. They are not merely mini-adults, for whom smaller films and less exposure are all that is required.

The differences occur under several headings as follows:

(1) conditions needing x-ray examination;
(2) anatomical proportions;
(3) exposure factors;
(4) radiation protection;
(5) methods of immobilization;
(6) co-operation.

CONDITIONS NEEDING X-RAY EXAMINATION

A good deal of adult pathology is not encountered in children. Conversely, many abnormal conditions are confined solely to childhood.

The first large group of these is the congenital abnormalities of the newborn which result in death if not treated. The whole field of medical and surgical treatment of the newborn has advanced greatly in recent years. Many infants now survive, who not so long ago would have died of their defects.

Atresias of the gastro-intestinal tract, severe congenital heart defects, hyaline membrane disease and other causes of the respiratory distress syndrome, spina bifida, bilateral choanal atresia, all present only in the first days of life.

Up to about the age of four years, malignant tumours of embryonic origin appear. These include neuroblastoma, nephroblastoma (Wilms' tumour) and others somewhat rarer.

There are infections which occur only in childhood, for instance croup.

Because of the different structure of a child's bones, the same injury to a child and an adult may have a different result. Only a child will sustain a greenstick fracture, or slipped epiphysis. Certain other ortho-paedic conditions, such as Perthes' disease of the hip, occur only in childhood. Congenital dislocation of the hips and talipes (club feet) are diagnosed and treated in infancy. Idiopathic scoliosis presents only in growing youngsters.

There are many other examples; there are also other conditions which are much commoner in children than in adults. A knowledge of these differences is important to a radiographer. Successful radiographic demonstration of any lesion is far easier if you know what you are aiming to show and the best projections for this purpose.

ANATOMICAL PROPORTIONS

The anatomical proportions of children are very different from those of an adult: the younger the child, the more marked the differences (Fig. I). A knowledge of where the chest ends and the abdomen begins in the body of an infant or child is essential for accurate positioning and field limitation. Only the area in question, and the *whole* of it, should appear on the radiograph.

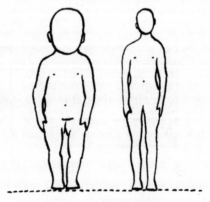

Fig. I.

The baby

The head is large in proportion to the body and the cranium to the face. The abdomen is large, the diaphragm high (Fig. 2).

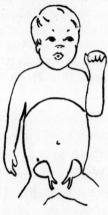

Fig. 2.

Kidneys are low, about midway between diaphragm and symphysis pubis, because of the large liver and stomach. The pelvic abdomen is tiny: the bladder extends above it. The chest, pelvis and limbs are small in proportion to the abdomen. The spine is straight at first: normal curves do not appear till the baby starts sitting upright. *Radiographically*, the important points are as follows.

Chest (Fig. 3)

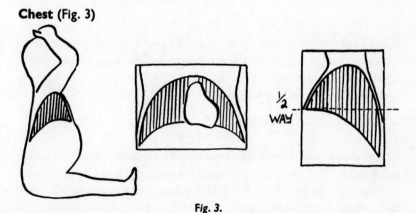

Fig. 3.

AP projection
The lungs appear wider than they are long and much higher up than you would think. The diaphragm is just below the level of the nipples. Use the cassette crosswise.

Lateral projection
The posterior part of the lungs may extend to *twice* the depth of the anterior part. Use the cassette lengthwise. Film size 13 × 18 cm (8 × 6 in) is used for infants; 18 × 24 cm (10 × 8 in) after about 6 months.

Abdomen
The measurements of length, width and depth in a given baby are much the same. A lateral view provides far more information than it would of a 6 or 7 year old, whose abdomen is comparatively flat. The abdomen bulges sideways wider than the pelvis (Fig. 4). This is not just fat, but

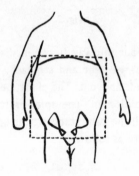

Fig. 4.

contains abdominal organs. So the bulge on each side must not be coned off by closing the light beam diaphragm to the edge of the pelvis. Over about 6 months, a 24 × 30 cm (12 × 10 in) film is needed to include the whole of the abdomen.

The toddler
All the above remarks still hold true but in a modified version. The head is full grown by 5 years, but the bones are not quite so dense as later on.

Size 18 × 24 cm (10 × 8 in) film will suffice for an infant's skull. Over about 8–9 months, a 24 × 30 cm (12 × 10 in) film is needed.

The child

From about 5 years the child starts to lose 'puppy-fat' and instead of being chubby can become quite skinny and tall by 7–8 years. After that some children run to fat again at the approach of adolescence. A 24 × 30 cm (12 × 10 in) cassette can still be used crosswise for a chest radiograph up to about 10 years.

EXPOSURE FACTORS

It will be obvious from all this that exposure factors do not vary by age-groups.

The skull exposure at 5 years is only very slightly less than for a teenager.

The chest exposure factors may be the same for a 2 or 3 year old and a 7 or 8 year old.

Unfortunately, it is not possible to give much detailed guidance on this subject, as there are so many variables involved. X-ray machines, films, screens, processing methods and radiologists' preferences vary from one department to another. All that can be done is to indicate a few general principles.

(i) Exposure time should be as short as possible, even with older children, to avoid movement blur.

(ii) The kilovoltage can be quite high, considering the thickness of a child compared with that of an adult: 60–65 kV for an infant's chest, 70–80 kV for an abdomen.

(iii) In a general hospital x-ray department, there should always be a chart of exposure factors for children in each room. This can be compiled by noting the factors used in every successful set of films taken of a child, with remarks as to age and build (e.g. small, fat 5 year old, very thin 10 year old, tiny premature infant, etc.). This helps others to adjust the factors for another patient, who may be the same age, but quite a different shape.

RADIATION PROTECTION

The patient

(1) The largest dose of unnecessary radiation to a patient is caused by a *repeat film*. Every possible precaution must be taken to ensure that the

first attempt produces a film of adequate diagnostic quality. If there is doubt on any point, show the film to the radiologist (or the doctor who requested it). Though the film may not be ideal, it may provide sufficient information. If so, you save the child from being irradiated a second time. For the same reason, an inexperienced young radiographer should not be left to x-ray a child on her own.

To avoid the necessity of a repeat you should:

(i)   use the correct exposure factors;
(ii) use the shortest possible time;
(iii) be sure the child is adequately immobilized.

(2) The *smallest possible area* should be irradiated, consistent with producing the necessary information. Far too large a field is often used, particularly in the case of babies. Arms and legs should not appear on an abdomen film, nor half the skull and abdomen on a chest film.

(3) *Lead gonad protection* should always be used. The only exception is when there is a possibility that it may obscure relevant detail. This arises in the case of a small girl's hips encased in a plaster spica, for example. If you cannot be absolutely sure of accurate placing of the lead, it is better not to risk having to repeat the film.

(4) *During fluoroscopy* a sheet of lead rubber should lie under a baby's pelvis except, of course, during enemas.

(5) The *routine number of views* necessary in any examination depends on the radiologist. In general hospitals it may be considered necessary to take more views than in a children's hospital as the radiologists may not be used to viewing children's radiographs.

(6) It is useful to note *exposure factors* (and which x-ray machine) on films of a child likely to have many follow-up films, especially if the pathology needs more or less than normal.

Adults holding patients

If certain precautions are strictly observed, the radiation dose received by an adult helper can be negligible.

(i)   Ascertain if the mother (or nurse) is pregnant.
(ii) The same nurse should not hold different babies on the same day.
(ii) It must be remembered that lead coats protect *only from scattered radiation*. The adult should not stand in the primary beam. For chest

radiography there should be added lead protection incorporated in the chest stand. If there is not, the lead coat must be at least 0·35 mm lead equivalent. This is adequate at 6-ft distance for up to 70 kV only. Above that, 0·5 mm lead equivalent is necessary.

(iv) The x-ray beam must be collimated to within the cassette edges.

(v) There is not much scatter from children, but an adult's *hands* can easily come within the field of primary radiation. It is very difficult to hold a child accurately in position when wearing lead gloves. Therefore it is the radiographer's responsibility to show nurse or mother how to hold and keep her hands out of the x-ray beam at the same time.

(vi) the light-beam must correspond accurately with the x-ray field.

The drawings are meant as a guide to correct positioning. In some an adult's hands are drawn apparently unprotected. If correct radiographic technique, as described above, is employed, dose estimates have shown that, for a baby's chest radiograph, the dose to the adult helper's hands is about 1 millirem. The maximum permissible dose (Table BII Code of Practice) for the extremities is 7·5 rems per year.

Old lead-rubber gloves can be cut up into various shapes for protection. One of the most useful can be made from the cuff. The cut-out bit allows the epiphysis to be seen (Fig. 5).

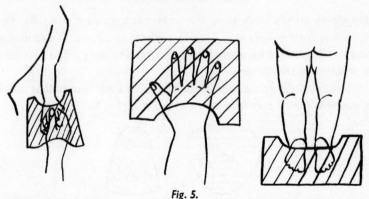

Fig. 5.

During fluoroscopy of a baby, a sheet of lead rubber should be carefully positioned each side of baby's head, under nurse's hands. It must not obscure the radiologist's view of baby swallowing. Nurse's hands, holding baby's arms up by his head and the feeding bottle, should never appear on the television screen.

Other people

Theatre work: any staff in the theatre during fluoroscopy, or when an x-ray exposure is made, must wear lead rubber coats.

Ward mobile examinations: these should be undertaken only if it is quite impossible to move the child (if necessary even in his bed) to the x-ray department.

All nurses, visiting mothers (who may be pregnant) and child patients up and about in the ward must be well out of the way before an x-ray exposure is made. Other children or babies in cots and incubators nearby should be moved if possible to 6-ft distance. Ask a nurse to watch out for little ones making a sudden dash in the wrong direction. Great care must be taken when using a horizontal beam. Look well beyond your patient, to make sure no child or adult is in line with the x-raybeam. Do not aim it at a thin partition wall.

X-ray staff

No radiographer, even in a lead coat, should hold a child for x-ray examination.

Lead-rubber cut-outs

Lead gloves usually crack along the creases at the side of the cuffs. Two cut-outs as described on page 7 can be cut from one glove. The remaining hand and fingers can be used to protect a hand holding a film vertically, for instance in the theatre.

Various sizes of gonad protection cut from 0·5 mm lead rubber should be available for all ages from birth to teenage (Fig. 6).

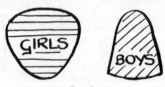

Fig. 6.

IMMOBILIZATION

Keeping still does not come naturally to small children. They move, sometimes even when trying their best not to. The avoidance of movement blur on radiographs is achieved in two ways: by speed and by adequate immobilization.

Speed

Short exposure times are essential: 0·02s maximum for chests, 0·04s for abdomens (unless the child is old enough to hold his breath). Consequently a high milliamperage, fast Potter Bucky and fine grids are needed. A focal spot of 0·1 mm² is satisfactory for general work. In the x-ray department of a general hospital there will be several different machines from which to choose in dealing with paediatric patients. Use whichever will provide the highest milliamperage. It is worth while asking the parents to wait a little, if necessary, if the room you want is in use at the time. Explain why and they will rarely object.

Two radiographers working together as a team, one to centre the tube and make the exposure, the other to position the child for mother to hold, will achieve results with far greater speed than two working separately. With experience, it is possible to develop a sort of 'snapshot' technique, where a child that is struggling is 'snapped' when momentarily in the right position. All children should be watched carefully immediately before the exposure is made.

Restraint

Babies keep still only when they are very ill. Otherwise they greatly resent being forcibly restrained, especially in an unusual position. Struggling is their only form of protest (apart from bawling!) and even tiny ones are quite surprisingly strong.

It is possible to restrain a baby or toddler completely with various combinations of Velcro straps, bandages and sandbags; but it will be found that these need to be so tight or heavy, if they are to be effective on their own, as to cause considerable distress and discomfort. Usually, a really determined struggler can squirm out of almost any restriction.

There are several immobilization devices, some quite complex, on the market. They may well be efficient but children photographed in them usually look anything but happy. Few of these devices will be found in use in children's hospitals. Most paediatric radiographers I have spoken to are agreed that the best method of immobilization is a pair of adult hands, adequately protected.

The next most widely used aid is the ordinary compression band, quick and easy to adjust, and available in all x-ray departments. It is used over the hips for examinations of the upper half of a child and across the chest for the lower half.

When using it across the hips, put a wedge-shaped foam pad under it, thin end towards the abdomen (Fig. 7). Otherwise the difference in thickness between abdomen and thighs causes the edge of the band to compress the abdomen uncomfortably when it is tightened.

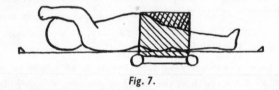

Fig. 7.

When using it across the chest, leave the arms free. Pinioning a toddler's arms to his sides will make him struggle to free them.

A small baby is most easily x-rayed just after a feed, if this can be arranged. He may then sleep peacefully and need no restraint apart from a sandbag each side to stop him rolling. The baby ward or mother can sometimes provide a dummy, which can prove invaluable in pacifying a crying infant.

A specially made stand (such as is illustrated in Chapter 2) for chest and erect abdomen examinations, is worth going to some trouble to acquire. It is the only completely satisfactory method of supporting a cassette vertically and immobilizing the baby for these examinations.

Breathing

The only time when it is advantageous to have a baby crying, is for x-ray examination of the chest. If you time the exposure correctly, you can then be sure of maximum inspiration.

Children over about 7 or 8 can hold their breath for an examination, but need to be carefully rehearsed several times beforehand. It can be confusing to ask them to stop breathing on *expiration*. This is necessary only when films must be taken on both inspiration and expiration.

For chest radiographs, make sure the shoulders do not rise as the child breathes in. For abdomen radiographs, tell him to take in only a small breath, and keep his tummy still.

Examinations of other parts of the body do not require the breath to be held.

CO-OPERATION

Small babies can be held still in position. School-age children will mostly do what is asked of them without a fuss. It is from about 8 or 9 months to about 5 years that difficulties in co-operation may arise. A little thought beforehand can save a lot of trouble.

Waiting

In a general x-ray department, a corner of the waiting-room should be specially equipped for children. If the number of child patients justifies it (or in an accident centre) a separate waiting-room of their own is better still. Brightly-coloured pictures or posters on the wall, a pile of comics and picture-books and a few toys, can make a lot of difference to a child's frame of mind when his turn comes to be x-rayed. Various soft toys, a plastic telephone, a nest of boxes, building blocks, some kind of small rocking-horse or other animal than can be sat upon, are recommended; jigsaws, squeaky or noisy toys and balls, are *not* advisable. Most hospitals have a League of Friends who would help in providing some of these.

Preparation of x-ray room

Read the request form carefully. If you have any queries as to the examination requested, now is the time to deal with them, not when the child is on the table. Decide on the views to be taken and get the right number of the right size cassette ready. Check that foam pads, lead protection, sandbags, and anything else you may need are at hand (and not being used by someone else in another room). Set the exposure approximately. If your patient is too young for explanations, run the anode so that the sudden noise of it starting to rotate won't distract or startle him once he is positioned. Lock the tube at the right height or distance. NEVER bring it closer to a child especially if he's lying on the table: this can be very frightening. Note the child's name on the form, including surname: parents also appreciate being addressed personally.

Choice of helper

Children over 5 or 6 will generally come quite happily when called, often by themselves. Younger ones will probably need the reassurance of a parent's presence. Never forget to enquire if a mother is pregnant. If so, she can take the child into the room first, then leave: father or a nurse must hold him. Toddlers often behave better with father anyway; if mother is not pregnant, leave the choice to the parents themselves. It is better to have only one of them, to start with at any rate. However, a bellowing, struggling, 2 year old may prove too much of a handful for one parent and need both to hold him still.

A mother should never be turned away at the door of the x-ray room and the child taken from her. It will only upset them both.

Approach to the child

You must always try to gain the trust and co-operation of your small patients; you should also be able to vary your technique so as to manage without. The following suggestions are based not only on my own experience but also on that of other paediatric radiographers in two children's hospitals. Others may disagree with these ideas: I do not claim that they are the only way but simply that they work.

Each child, of any age, is a separate individual personality. The following remarks are to be read as generalizations only, not as dogmatic statements. The division into age-groups is purely arbitrary and to be taken just as a rough guide. It is based on the supposition that, generally speaking, over 3 years explanations will be at least partly understood, under 3 years, probably not.

6 months–$2\frac{1}{2}$ to 3 years

Mother should sit baby on the x-ray table to undress him, while you explain to her what you are going to do. Talk to the child also: though the words won't be understood, the tone of voice conveys a great deal. Put the lead coat on mother as she stands beside the child. Distract his attention with a squeaky rubber toy, or a music box. Once you've got his attention, the toy can be placed in a strategic position so that he will look in the right direction.

Do not take a child over 6 months or so away from mother in the mistaken belief you can 'make friends' with him. Some won't mind; some will start bawling—there is no way of telling beforehand. The ones you upset are going to be more difficult to x-ray, so it is safer not to risk it. Do not leave a baby alone on the table: he can easily roll off.

If baby starts crying, just carry on and get the examination over as quickly as you can.

Resistance (same age)
If a child under 3 years decides to resist being x-rayed, it is no good trying to reason, insist or distract. None will work, you are only wasting time.

Regrettably, force must be used for restraint, and the quicker you get on with it the better. Borrow a nurse from the out-patient department or the ward. It is almost impossible to determine whether a resistant 1–2 year old is motivated by fear or temper: the mother is your only guide. If she thinks he's frightened, explain quickly and clearly what you want her to do, get him in position, and ask mother and nurse to hold him firmly there. Don't strap him down with Velcro or compression band. If she says its pure temper, ask her to leave the room (she will probably be quite glad to) and immobilize him with the aid of nurse and one or even two compression bands. Get it all over as quickly as possible and restore him immediately to mother.

Keep talking to the child as you position him (if you can be heard!) in a *calm, friendly* tone.

In a case like this, two radiographers can work together as a team to great advantage. One positions the child, and changes the cassettes. The other centres the tube, and makes the exposure (see p. 28).

3–5 years
There should be a chair just inside the door of the x-ray room, where mother can sit down with the child on her lap. Explain to him that you are going to take his photograph with a special 'camera'. Use a friendly but firm tone of voice. It is well worth while spending some time trying

to gain his interest and attention at this point. Speak directly to him, call him by name. Ask *him* the questions even when mother keeps answering for him. Explain about the 'camera', demonstrate the light beam diaphragm ('this is the light that will take your picture, it can make itself big and small'), let him look at it close up if he wants to. Demonstrate a shadow of your hand on the x-ray table. Run the anode, tell him that the 'buzzy' noise is all that is going to happen. Small children are not usually scared by all the machinery; more often they are quite interested.

Children over 3 will mostly understand what is required of them. Don't go into long explanations, be brief and simple. Don't say 'It won't hurt'—the thought may not have crossed his mind.

If it *is* going to hurt (moving a fractured limb, or an intravenous injection) do not ever lie about it. A child who suffers pain after being told he won't, will never believe such reassurance again.

If the examination consists of several projections, start with whichever is easiest for the child: a lateral chest before a PA view, a post-nasal space before an occipito-mental view for sinuses.

Frightened 3–5 years

The emotionally insecure child, or one who has had a previous frightening experience of hospital, will make difficulties at the start. If he clings and cries and makes a fuss, don't take him away from his mother. He is better sitting on a chair by himself, while you help her into a lead coat.

If he seems frightened, try to get him to tell you why; it may be just one small thing, easily rectified. Little ones' fears can seem quite irrational. It may be lying down, or having his jersey taken off, the feel of a cold cassette, or just the shape of something in the room. One small boy was quite happy until a piece of lead rubber protection was placed on him: it terrified him. Another could not be persuaded to extend his (uninjured) arm; careful questioning finally revealed he was afraid of an injection if he did. The approach of someone in a white coat is enough to frighten some children.

If he is clutching a toy, or even a piece of material (which may be a precious 'comforter') don't take it away. Teddy or Panda can have his 'picture' taken too, with a little ingenuity in positioning.

Flexibility of technique is essential: if a child will not be positioned in one way, try another. If he refuses to lie down on the table, an erect film is often possible. If he won't put his arm on the table perhaps he will stand in front of the chest stand.

A really terrified child can watch from the safety of mother's arms (behind a lead screen through a lead glass window) another child having a simple examination, such as a hand or chest x-rayed.

Sedation is a last resort. It is far better to try to remove the cause of fear and convince the child there is nothing to be scared about.

Spoilt 3–5 years

Only experience will teach you how to distinguish between a spoilt and a frightened child, when you are faced with defiance right from the start. Instant judgments, of a 'spoilt brat' and a 'hopeless' mother can quite easily be mistaken. It is wiser to begin by assuming that a 3 or 4 year old's flat refusal to be examined may be prompted by fear. Ask mother if she knows of any possible cause. He may have unpleasant memories of a previous visit to hospital. (Regrettably, he may even have been bullied or frightened in an x-ray department.)

Even if it seems he is just spoilt and wilful, treat him at first as you would any other child. Indicate by your tone and manner that you expect him to do what he's told, but keep your voice matter-of-fact and friendly. Ask mother to get him ready. It will shortly become obvious whether he usually gets his own way or not. The mother who pleads 'Do be a good boy, darling, just to please mummy' is almost invariably answered 'No, don't *want* to!'

When it is apparent to mother that she is getting nowhere, suggest he might behave better if you got a nurse to hold him while she leaves the room. Either she will accept your suggestion gladly, or she will ask the child if that is what he would prefer—whereupon his resistance will probably vanish at the mere idea.

You should not threaten the child yourself with substituting a nurse for his mother if he isn't 'good'. Don't get exasperated, no matter what the provocation. Don't let it become a long drawn-out battle of wills. If you see you are losing, keep calm and alter your tactics. Get another radiographer to come and assist you. Remember it is not your job to teach the child a lesson in discipline, however much you may be tempted. It is simply to x-ray him.

On the other hand, if you appear to give in, and try coaxing, he will sense at once that he is winning, and become more adamant than ever.

If he is absolutely impossible, tell mother and child that you are too busy to wait any longer, that you will go away to x-ray another little boy (or girl) and to call you back when he's ready to co-operate. Explain to mother that the only alternative is an appointment on another day, and sedation; that it will take several hours then as against a few minutes now. Then leave them alone for five minutes or so. This almost always works (bribery probably does the trick). If it doesn't, sedation is the only answer.

It is much better to give up and try again another day, than to go on taking several useless films. By persevering you will only irradiate him to no purpose and ensure that he will never willingly enter an x-ray department again.

Over 5 years
Normal school-age children rarely refuse to co-operate. Even those who cause problems to parents or teachers, or the nurses in the ward, often behave perfectly for the short time they are in the x-ray department.

Older children who appear babyish, by thumbsucking or carrying a doll or animal toy into the x-ray room with them, should not be humiliated by having remarks made about this.

Occasionally a 6 or 7 year old may be hiding the fact that he is frightened. One small patient burst into tears, from relief *after* the examination, which he had endured apparently quite cheerfully. A child under perhaps 8 or 9 should not be left alone on the x-ray table: there should be a relative or nurse with him. If he has to lie there for some time, for instance during excretion urography, give him a few comics. A book requires too much concentration.

Never lie to a child, of any age. Don't say the examination is nearly over when it is only just started. Don't say a painful procedure won't hurt. When an appointment is made for excretion urography, micturating cystogram or barium enema, the parent should be warned, preferably out of hearing of the child, exactly what is entailed. The decision to tell the child then, or leave it to the day of the examination, should be left to the parent. However, just before any unpleasant experience, the child must be told what is going to happen. Any questions must be answered truthfully.

If he hasn't been warned about an injection beforehand, don't tell him until the doctor has actually arrived in the department. Sometimes there can be quite a delay before a house-surgeon is available, long enough for a child to get quite worked-up. Ask the doctor if he would prefer to tell the child himself.

During the injection, mother or a nurse should stand on the opposite side of the table from the doctor and distract the child by talking about something else.

School-age children, particularly little girls, are often very shy about undressing in public. It is useful to have a supply of small x-ray gowns, or dressing gowns. If there are none, the child should undress in the x-ray room, not in a cubicle. Don't leave the door wide open. Cover the child with a blanket on the x-ray table. Expose only the area to be x-rayed. Don't leave a child lying half-naked on the table before a micturating cystogram or barium enema.

An injured child of any age should never be left alone.

Sedation

Emotionally maladjusted children of school age and those who are unnaturally apprehensive, or who have had a previous unpleasant experience of hospitals, may need sedation. This should be discussed with the referring doctor and/or the parents beforehand. The radiologist will decide on the type and the dosage.

In some x-ray departments, children under 5 or 6 are routinely sedated for excretion urography. In others, it is not considered advantageous, in that a sedated child becomes irritable when disturbed and may resist the injection even more strenuously than if he were awake. Sedation is usually considered helpful for catheterization for a micturating cystogram even on older children, but in this case they may have to be examined supine instead of in the usuall erect position. The decision rests with the radiologist who is to perform the examination.

Parents

Mothers need some thought and kindness also. They are naturally anxious, especially if it is a first visit to hospital. Mothers of very new babies are especially vulnerable. Explain that it isn't really cruel to strap tiny ones down with Velcro and ignore their crying when position-ing, even though it may appear so. Always restore an infant or young child to mother for comforting the moment you have finished taking your film. It is unkind to keep a crying baby immobilized on the table, just for your own convenience, while a film is being processed. Pick him up yourself and comfort him while mother takes off the lead coat, holding baby facing mother so that he can see she is still there.

Parents often need reassurance about radiation protection. They wonder, since *they* have to be protected, what harm is being done to their child. Explain that it has been considered necessary that the child should be x-rayed, but not that they should be. Parents of children who have many x-ray examinations tend to get worried about this and will ask for gonad protection to be used if they think it is being omitted. Their wishes must be respected and one should try not to be irritated at being told one's job. The protection may have been left off on a previous occasion; the parents are only trying to safeguard their own child.

Be careful what you say aloud in the hearing of waiting parents. You may be talking to another member of staff about a different child, but parents are apt to think theirs is the only one in the department and may be alarmed by what they overhear. If a child has to return for a follow-up examination (for instance, of the chest after an infection), reassure the parents that it is not because something serious has been found wrong with him.

If a mother stays with a child during an injection for excretion urography, keep an eye on her. She may appear to be perfectly all right, and then quite suddenly faint, or get upset. You must act quickly to get her out of the child's sight before she does either, so be alert to warning signs. A mother with a badly-injured child is often better left outside the room during the examination: she will be emotionally upset anyway by the shock of his injury and the child should not see her in tears.

Finally, when a child of any age leaves the x-ray department, his experience should have been such that he will not mind if he ever has to come again. Spend a minute or two chatting to him before he leaves to make certain that, even if he was scared before, he is now reassured.

No child should ever dread a return visit to an x-ray department because of bad handling on a previous occasion.

SOME ACCESSORIES

Essential items

Compression band (two if possible)
Strips of Velcro, different lengths
Strips of clear film (for hands) 6 cm wide
Lengths of orthopaedic flannel bandage (lateral skull, etc.)
Sandbags
Different sizes and shapes of foam pads; small pieces of foam
Squeaky rubber toy (for distracting attention)
Baby chest stand
Toddler seat for chest examination } see Chapter 2

Additional useful items

Comics for various ages
Picture story-books
Small number of safe, simple toys
Coloured pictures or transfers stuck on wall or equipment in suitable
    place for the child to keep his eyes on when positioned
Music box (for distraction of babies)
Tubular elasticated bandage 10 cm (4 in) wide (for restraint of babies'
legs)
Jelly babies (for bribery!)

Lead protection

Small lead rubber shapes (not less than 0·5 mm) for gonad protection
Pieces of lead rubber cut from cuffs of old gloves to protect adult hands
    (see Fig. 5, p. 7)
Lead gloves for use in holding cassettes, or supporting a child upright
Larger rectangular pieces of lead rubber (0·5 mm) for shielding parts of
    body from primary radiation, and adults' hands in fluoroscopy of
    infants
Lead rubber apron with Velcro straps for use in chest radiography
    (also to protect body in certain positions for radiography of the arm)

CHAPTER 2
THE CHEST

Chest radiography constitutes by far the greatest part of all radiography of children. The younger the child the more difficult it is to take a really good radiograph.

The standard views in any hospital are, of course, determined by the radiologist. Some require erect PA projections at all ages, even the newborn. In some hospitals an AP projection is acceptable up to the age of sitting unsupported. Where no special cassette holder for erect radiography of babies is available, AP supine films are usual.

Again, the routine lateral view is omitted in some hospitals, or is taken only if the AP or PA film shows some abnormality. When a cardiac clinic is held at intervals in the out-patient department, it may be routine for all children attending to have a PA film taken on arrival, and further views later at the request of the cardiologist.

Generally it is better to remove all upper clothing for the examination, as the kilovoltage range employed is low. Vest or pyjama tops may cause lines to appear over the lung fields. Exceptions may occasionally be made, and a vest left on if it is wool or cotton. It is not worth while having a battle of wills with a 3 year old who refuses to part with his vest, but make a note on the request form for the radiologist's information. The cold front of the cassette can be covered with a paper towel. Long hair, especially plaits, should be pinned up or hung over the back of the cassette.

If a child is likely to have several follow-up films taken at brief intervals for the same condition, the exposure factors should be noted on the first occasion and used for all subsequent films so that the series is consistent for comparison. If a child's first x-ray examination is to consist of PA and lateral views, take the lateral view first; it is more reassuring for him.

Chest radiography of newborn infants is described in Chapter 12.

RADIOGRAPHIC TECHNIQUE

Older children (school age)

The older child, from 6 years or so on, rarely presents difficulties and will normally stand for the examination. There are two important points.

Breathing

Rehearse the child in holding his breath. Often children will breathe *out* again immediately after breathing in. If he is only 5 years old and finds it difficult, do not let him get flustered about it. Just ask him to breathe in and, watching him carefully, expose just as he reaches full inspiration.

Erect posture

Especially in the lateral position, with the arms folded over the top of the head, most children tend to stoop with head bent forward. Make sure the back is straight and head erect, to expand the chest.

Routine views

PA view

Position the child with chest against the cassette, chin on the top edge. Arms are either around it, hugging it to him, or folded over the top of

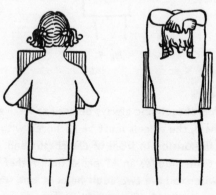

Fig. 8.

his head with elbows forward. The shoulders must not hunch up towards the ears. A small lead-rubber apron with Velcro straps is useful for immobilization as well as protection, if the chest stand is such that the straps can go round it as well as the child's waist (Fig. 8). Centre to the centre of the cassette, not the 4th dorsal vertebra. Limit the field to within the edges of the cassette. A 24 × 30 cm (12 × 10 in) cassette can be used crosswise up to about 10 years. This ensures that the name space does not appear over the apex of one lung.

Lateral view
The film is used in the normal vertical position in the cassette holder. The arms should be crossed over the head, hands holding the opposite elbows (Fig. 9). Check that the rib-cage is correctly aligned at right angles to the cassette, as it is easy for this view to turn out slightly oblique. Centre to the centre of the cassette.

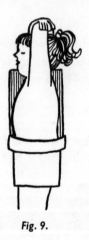

Fig. 9.

Stretcher patients
A stretcher with brakes should always be used to fetch a child from the ward. Lacking them, the wheels must be anchored with sandbags when the stretcher is in position in front of the chest stand. Sometimes it is easier to support the child for an AP projection, rather than a PA, if he is very ill. It is wiser to have two adult helpers, one standing each side of the child. A limp, ill, 10–12 year old is more than one person can

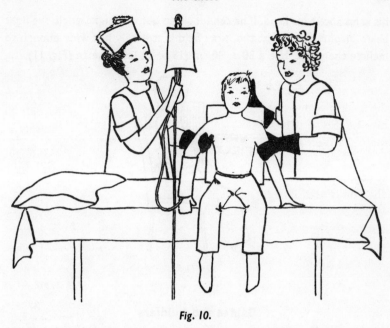

Fig. 10.

manage alone, and there may be an intravenous drip to watch out for also (Fig. 10).

Chair patients
A child too shaky to stand must be x-rayed sitting down, but a wheelchair is highly unsuitable for radiography. A firm metal-framed chair with a broad flat seat is ideal and it requires little effort to transfer the child on to it.

PA view
Seat him sideways on the chair so that the chairback is to one side of the chest-stand. Ask him to put his arms round the cassette. A nurse should hold him if he needs support. In this case, he folds his arms over his head, elbows forward; and nurse, standing at the side, can hold his upper arms.

Lateral view
Change his position on the seat so that his back is to the chair back, with two rectangular foam pads between. Nurse stands facing him and holds

his arms above his head. If he cannot sit up quite straight, angle the light beam diaphragm so that the x-ray field is still only just wide enough to include the chest. Use a 30 × 40 cm (15 × 12 in) cassette (Fig. 11).

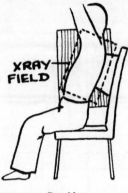

Fig. 11.

Babies and toddlers

It is in the age-group between infants and school-age that the greatest difficulties arise, both in positioning and co-operation (or lack of it). The following sub-divisions are quite arbitrary but are useful as a rough guide to suitable techniques at different ages.

Babies and small children's lungfields are wider than they are long in the AP and PA projections. Use the cassette crosswise. In the lateral projection, the posterior lung bases may be as much as twice the depth of the anterior lung, so open the light beam diaphragm accordingly, and use the cassette vertically (Fig. 12).

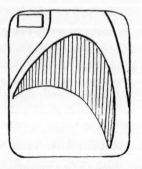 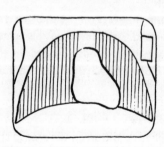

Fig. 12.

1–6 months

Good radiographs of these babies in the erect position are almost impossible without a special cassette holder. A simple wooden one, as in Fig. 13, is easily made by the hospital carpenters and can stand on the end of the x-ray table. Flat wooden bars, of varying height, which fit in the slots of the uprights and rest on the crossbar, provide an easy way

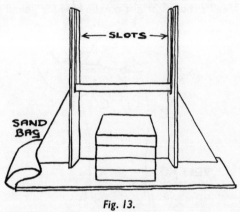

Fig. 13.

of raising the height of the cassette. Foam pads, of varying thicknesses to cover the seat, do the same for the height of the baby. Velcro is stuck all around the sides of the seat. A Velcro strap can then be placed across a baby's thighs at any angle. Ideally there should also be a sheet of lead-ply, or lead rubber, at the back of this stand. However, if this is difficult to incorporate, the nurse or mother holding the baby is adequately protected providing she is wearing a coat of *not less than 0·5 mm* lead equivalent. This is effective for even primary radiation at the low kilo-voltages used for babies' chests. A sandbag is placed each side of the stand.

Erect AP or PA view

Put a cassette in the holder, covered with a paper towel. Place baby sitting astride the seat. Nurse stands behind the chest stand and holds baby without raising his arms. Fasten the Velcro strap across his thighs (but not on bare skin: Velcro can mark a baby's skin quite badly. Use a folded paper towel to prevent this). Make sure he is sitting straight.

Raise the arms gently, and slowly, bringing the elbows forward first, each side of the face, not out sideways from the body. Babies hate having their arms extended and resist with surprising strength. The arms should not be extended fully, as this causes baby to lean backwards. Nurse holds the head and arms together, with her index fingers on baby's forehead (AP position) or occiput (PA position) (Fig. 14). She should exert a slight pull upwards, to ensure baby is not 'slumping'. Prop a small piece of lead rubber upright on the seat for gonad protection.

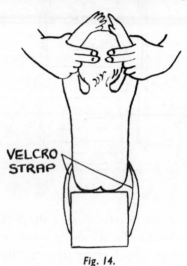

VELCRO STRAP

Fig. 14.

AP. If baby is struggling, it is very easy for nurse to put her finger in his eye, so warn her!

PA. As a baby's neck is very short it is not possible to put the chin on the top edge of the cassette, or the lung apices will not be on the radiograph. The correct height for the cassette is such that his nose and mouth are at the level of the edge. Great care is needed on nurse's part to see his face is not damaged if he struggles.

Erect lateral view

Place baby sitting sideways to the cassette. Strap his thighs as before. Nurse holds his left arm with her left hand, his right arm with her right. Her wrist will then be behind his head and will stop him throwing it backwards and arching his back (Fig. 15).

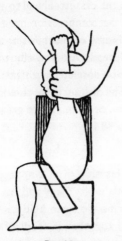

Fig. 15.

There may be a polythene tube emerging from one of baby's nostrils, then stuck to the side of his face with sticky tape, leaving a length of several inches dangling free and spigotted at the end. This is a naso-gastric feeding tube and will appear only on a baby coming from the ward. The tubing is radio-opaque, so it should always be hung over the back of the cassette, out of the way.

Supine AP view

Place the cassette in position near one end of the x-ray table. Raise the top edge of it on an inch thick piece of foam which also serves to cushion baby's head. This prevents the projection from being lordotic. Centre the x-ray beam to the cassette, cone within its edges and cover it with a

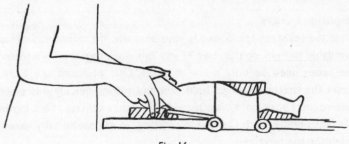

Fig. 16.

paper towel. Lay baby on the cassette, head towards the end of the table, on the foam pad. Adjust the compression band across the pelvis, with a foam pad underneath it. Nurse or mother stands at the end of the table, holding baby's arms and head with the elbows flexed against the ears (Fig. 16). The head must be *absolutely straight*: that is, exactly as for an AP view of the skull. The distance routinely used is decided by the radiologist. It may be 36 in. or 40 in. or the greatest height obtainable on the tube column (usually 48 in).

Lateral view
The baby is turned on his side. The compression band is again used across the pelvis but with a 45° foam pad each side of baby, to avoid rotation (Fig. 17). The arms are again held each side of the face, beside the ears. If they are held together in front of the face, the thorax will rotate forwards, resulting in an oblique view.

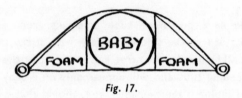

Fig. 17.

Ideally, these films should all be taken on full inspiration. With a crying baby this is simple enough. Watch carefully for a moment or two, with the anode rotating. You can then judge the length of a yell and anticipate the gasp of breath at the end of it. If he is not crying, you must watch the movement of the abdomen: it *protrudes* with the descent of the diaphragm on inspiration. A very short exposure time (0·02 s at most) is essential.

6 months–3 years
This is the resistant age. Speed is your best ally. If a second radiographer is available to help, so that two of you can work together as a team, the time taken need be only a few minutes. One positions the baby, instructs the mother how to hold him and moves quickly out of range when correct positioning is achieved. The other centres the x-ray beam and stands ready, with the anode rotating, to expose as baby takes in a breath for the next yell.

These children should ideally be x-rayed in the PA erect position. Although a 18 × 24 cm (10 × 8 in) film used crosswise is still large enough, it is better to use a 24 × 30 cm (12 × 10 in) size for a 2–3 year old: positioning has to be very exact with the smaller size film. If AP supine chest radiographs of this age-group are acceptable in your hospital, proceed as described above for the younger baby. If the radiologist wishes the films to be taken erect, some method of immobilizing the child must be arranged. It is easier to keep him still and straight in a sitting position.

A baby's high-chair or a four-legged wooden stool of the old-fashioned kind can be adapted for this purpose, with the aid of the hospital carpenters. The high-chair back is sawn off. A wooden platform is attached across the bottom rungs, strong enough to hold as many sandbags as the department can provide. A Velcro strap is attached to the seat, glued right across underneath it. Another can be attached to the front legs (Fig. 18). There should be no foot-rest so as to discourage efforts at standing up. It is used in conjunction with the adult chest stand.

Whatever is adapted for this purpose, whether stool, table or high-chair, it is important to bear in mind that toddlers are incredibly strong and can be very determined in their resistance. So the seat must be as solid as a rock, or there is a risk of the whole lot tipping over.

With the child in position for PA, AP or lateral projection, the technique for holding the arms and head is the same as described for

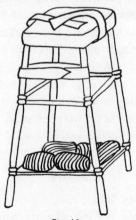

Fig. 18.

babies. The arms are held by the elbows. It may be found that father, or a really strong nurse, is more efficient at this job than mother.

On the less frequent occasions when you encounter no difficulty, it may not be necessary to use the Velcro strapping. The child's elbows should be held firmly in the same way, but, for the lateral view, mother can stand facing him. She can then engage his attention so that he keeps looking at her, instead of over his shoulder to see what you are doing.

3–5 years

From about 3 years on, a child may well co-operate, and can stand for the examination. However, in most departments an x-ray tube cannot be brought down low enough to use a horizontal beam at the height of a 3 year old. He will have to stand on a step, or a wooden box. There is no hope of getting a child of this age to hold his breath. See if he will just breathe in when you ask him, without hunching up his shoulders. If he gets bothered about this, it is better not to persist. Just watch his breathing when he is positioned, and expose on normal inspiration.

An ill child of this age is best x-rayed sitting down.

Radiation protection

(1)   Small lead-rubber aprons, which are obtainable in several sizes, should be used if available.

Small sitting patients can have a piece of lead rubber propped up with a sandbag in the appropriate position.

(2)   The adult holding a child from behind a chest stand is in direct line with the primary beam. Lead-rubber coats must not be less than 0·35 mm lead equivalent. A fixed lead screen gives still better protection. It is often not possible to hold correctly wearing lead rubber gloves. Therefore, it is the responsibility of the radiographer to ensure that a nurse's hands are outside the field of primary radiation.

(3)   Close the light beam diaphragm to within the cassette edges.

Faults

(1)   **Too large an x-ray field**.

A baby's chest radiograph not infrequently includes all or part of the skull, the abdomen, and adult hands. This is usually caused by ignorance of how small in area a baby's lungfields are. Looking at the drawings in the section on 'proportion' in Chapter I (pp. 2, 3) should help to overcome this error.

(2) **Rotation**

The inner ends of the clavicles must be equidistant from the spine on the radiograph. Even a very small degree of rotation, hardly noticeable in an adult, will produce an oblique projection of a baby's chest. The commonest cause is the head not being held strictly straight. It is most important that AP and PA projections should be *exactly* AP or PA. Rotation can lead to a variety of mis-diagnoses.

(3) **Lordosis**

It is very difficult to avoid a lordotic projection, both AP and PA. The 'bucket-handle' effect, when the anterior rib-ends appear turned up

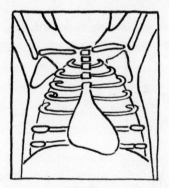

Fig. 19.

above the level of the corresponding posterior parts (Fig. 19) is due to bad positioning. It is caused by the following:

(i)   baby's feet being on the same level as his bottom: sit him on a seat;

(ii)   arms being fully extended, making him lean backwards: do not extend them;

(iii)   AP, baby 'slumping' (Fig. 20): nurse should exert a slight pull upwards as she holds baby;

PA, the normal protruding abdomen (Fig. 21): he must be held leaning slightly forwards;

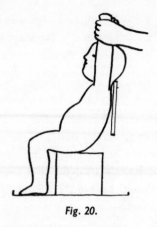

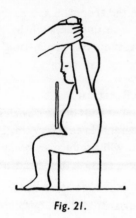

Fig. 20.   Fig. 21.

(iv)   a resistant toddler:

PA, throwing his head backwards and arching his back (Fig. 22): adult's
fingers must encircle the back of his head to prevent this, all the fingers
if necessary;

AP, lifting his bottom and leaning backwards (Fig. 23): correct use of
Velcro strapping stops this.

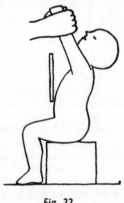

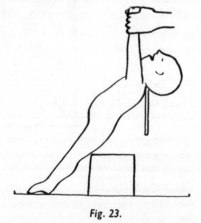

Fig. 22.   Fig. 23.

The object of Velcro strapping in either projection is to prevent
the child from standing up or slumping down, and to anchor his pelvis
firmly parallel to the cassette. (It must be tight.) The correct angle can
be seen in Fig. 24. If baby's thighs are bare, put a folded paper towel
under the strap.

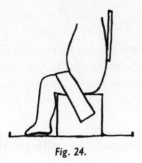

Fig. 24.

If the radiologist has no objection, tilting the x-ray tube 2°–5° downwards in the AP projection is helpful.

At least one-third of the total lung area in the AP view is obscured by the diaphragm. If, in addition, the projection is lordotic, an even larger area disappears. A posterior basal consolidation is, therefore, easily hidden.

(4) Motional blurring

The shortest possible exposure time, and a careful watching of the child's respiration rate before exposing, should eliminate blur caused by breathing or heartbeat. To deal with movement of the child himself, see section on 'immobilization' in Chapter I (p. 8).

(5) Expiration

There can be quite a striking difference between chest radiographs of a child taken on full inspiration and on expiration. It is possible to 'see' non-existent pathology on an expiration film. If only seven posterior ribs appear above the diaphragm on a PA or AP view, this warrants a repeat attempt. On full inspiration, eight or nine ribs can be counted above the diaphragm.

(6) Apices obscured or cut-off

The name-space will almost always be superimposed over a lung apex if the cassette is used vertically for an AP or PA projection. Putting a baby's chin on the top edge of a cassette when positioning for a PA view will result in the apices being off the film. Babies' necks are too short for this.

When positioning for an erect film, the height of both the x-ray tube and the cassette have to be adjusted to the patient, so it is not possible to set up everything ready beforehand. With the child seated in front of the cassette, adjust the film to the correct height, and centre to the centre of the cassette. Check the centring and coning again when the arms are raised.

Ward examination with mobile unit

A child who is unconscious, infectious, on traction or otherwise immobilized in bed, may have to be x-rayed in the ward. The request is not as frequent as in an adult hospital, because even very ill children can often be carried, or transported in the bed, to the x-ray department without harm.

The mobile machine used to x-ray a child's chest must be capable of giving 0·02-s exposure time and at least 200 mA. It is advisable to take an AP view only. The focal-film distance for supine radiography is, of course, limited to the height of the tube column and should be standardized on the exposure chart for all chest radiographs.

In a humidity tent (Croupette, Humidaire, etc.)

A child with asthma, croup or other similar condition may be in a polythene tent for oxygen and/or humidity therapy (Fig. 25). Ask the ward sister if you may open the front flap of this to take the film,

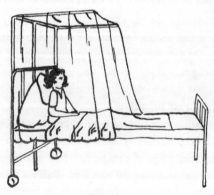

Fig. 25.

if the child is sitting up in bed. If you may, then prop a 30 × 40 cm (15 × 12 in) cassette vertically behind him with pillows and use a horizontal beam. Be as quick as you can, once you have opened the tent.

If the child is lying down, x-ray him supine through the roof of the tent. Being polythene, it is radio-translucent. Increase the kilovoltage by perhaps 2 or 3 kV. Try to avoid any creases or folds in the polythene, as they will cause lines on the radiograph. There may be a metal bar of the supporting frame to be avoided also. Small tents, for use with cots, are not supported by rigid bars, and will be too full of creases for this technique. They have to be folded back out of the way.

On a respirator
There will always be a nurse 'specialling' an unconscious child on a respirator. She will help you to get the cassette underneath the child. If there is a sandbag under the shoulders, substitute a foam pad. Do not move the head into the AP position yourself: nurse should do this. A sandbag will stop the head from rolling back to one side. Watch the rise and fall of the rib-cage carefully for a few minutes before you take the film. You can then judge the exact moment of full inspiration.

Under-water seal
Injury to the chest can result in air and/or blood leaking into the pleural space. (The same can happen after a thoracotomy, but chest surgery of children is not usually undertaken in a general hospital.) The treatment is insertion of a drainage tube connected to an underwater seal. This is a glass wide-necked jar, stoppered by a wide cork, having a long and short glass tube inserted through it. Water in the jar covers the long tube to a depth of an inch or so. The short tube acts as an air escape. One end of the drainage tube is sutured into the pleural space. The other end is attached by an airtight connection to the upper end of the long glass tube. Once connected to the child in his bed, the jar is placed on the floor under the bed. Fluid in the pleural space trickles down into the jar. Air in the pleural space is forced down the tube each time the child breathes in and it bubbles up through the water in the jar. Eventually all the air is expelled, and the lung re-expanded.

The jar must not be raised off the floor

The chest is x-rayed daily to assess re-expansion of the lung. Rehearse the child in as full an inspiration as he can manage and in holding his breath. Ask for a nurse to help you position him and get the cassette under or behind him. Take great care not to knock the jar accidentally, or pull on the drainage tube, in doing this.

PATHOLOGY

Diseases and infection of lungs

Acute bronchitis

Acute bronchitis usually occurs up to about 5 years of age: inflammation of the bronchi, with fever, cough and breathlessness.

Croup

Croup is an acute laryngitis, caused by a virus, occurring mainly between 6 months and 4 years. Breathing is difficult and accompanied by *stridor*, a hoarse whooping noise.

There is a very dangerous variety of croup, occurring in slightly older children, about 2–7 years. Not only the larynx is inflamed, but in particular the *epiglottis*. The child's condition can quite rapidly deteriorate to obstruction of the larynx, collapse and death. It can be a matter of grave urgency that the child is intubated by an anaesthetist to enable breathing to continue until the infection has subsided. Sometimes a tracheostomy is performed.

Acute bronchiolitis

Acute bronchiolitis occurs mainly in infants under 6 months. It is a viral infection causing inflammation of the bronchioles.

Pneumonia

Pneumonia is an infection of the alveoli of the lungs, occurring at any age, resulting in consolidation of lobules, a segment or an entire lobe of the affected lung. In infants there may be widespread small areas of consolidation. In school-age children the consolidation is more likely to be confined to one lobe. Lateral radiographs will show the exact location and extent of an area of consolidation, which may not be at all clearly visualized on the PA view.

Tuberculosis
Tuberculosis is a chronic infection which is now uncommon in Britain but tending to appear again in areas with a large immigrant population.

Asthma
Asthma is quite common in children. Over a period of time the chest grows barrel-shaped, the diaphragm becomes flattened (very noticeable in a lateral view) and the lungs emphysematous. Because of the over aeration of the lungs, the exposure factors need to be lower than normal—about 5 kV less—otherwise the films will be overexposed, and lung detail lost.

Cystic fibrosis
Lung symptoms appear eventually in cystic fibrosis, a congenital disease of the pancreas. From the radiographic point of view, the effect is the same as in asthma: hyper-aerated lungs needing less exposure. Radiographs of the sinuses are usually taken also, for initial diagnosis, as they are frequently opaque.

Metastases
Most childhood malignancies metastasize to the lungs. After surgical removal or treatment of a primary malignant growth, chest radiographs are taken at intervals.

Stridor
Stridor is not a disease, it is a symptom. It means the harsh grating sounds made by breathing when something is obstructing the larynx or trachea. The obstruction may be caused by:
(i)   inflammation, as for instance in croup;
(ii)   a foreign body inhaled and lodged in the upper airways;
(iii) something outside the larynx causing pressure: an anatomical abnormality in an infant; or, in the older baby, a swallowed foreign body lodged in the oseophagus.

Because of the varied causes of stridor, it is usual to take *a lateral view of the neck* in all cases of suspected croup, as well as the chest film.

Inhaled foreign bodies

Small objects are easily inhaled, by far the commonest being a peanut. Because of its shape and smoothness, it can travel quite a long way down the respiratory tract before becoming lodged. Small pieces of peanut can go even further. An opaque foreign body is easily seen on a radiograph. A non-opaque one, such as a peanut, can be localized only by demonstration of an area of collapse in the lung, or alternatively an area of greater translucency on expiration. The latter results from air being able to be breathed in past the obstruction, but its exit being blocked.

Consequently, PA or AP films on full inspiration and expiration may be essential for the radiological localization of the site of obstruction. This is not easy in the case of a baby or small child but every effort must be made to obtain these films none the less, as the removal of the obstructing foreign body may be a matter of urgency. The blocking of a bronchus needs immediate treatment. Even if only a small segment of lung is affected, the result may be a lung abscess if it is left untreated.

Fluids may be accidentally inhaled by children, causing inflammation of lung tissue. Examples are: the inhalation of milk, or vomit, by babies; of water in bathing accidents; or paraffin, bleach and other household poisons which small children may attempt to drink, choke on, and consequently inhale. All will need chest radiographs to assess the extent of damage and subsequent recovery.

Disorders of the pleural space

Pneumothorax, *haemothorax* and *pleural effusion* can all follow injury to the chest. Pleural effusion is also caused by inflammation of the lung from infection, or may develop above the site of a sub-phrenic abscess.

The spontaneous pneumothorax which occurs in adults is found occasionally in teenagers. In younger children, pneumothorax from any cause is very rare but may occur with haemothorax after injury to the chest wall in a road accident.

Pneumothorax may also be present in a newborn infant.

If there is difficulty in demonstrating any of these conditions radiographically in routine projections, or if the child is too ill for erect films, they can be shown by decubitus techniques using a horizontal beam.

Fluid in the pleural cavity: a small thick foam mattress, or enough foam pads of the same size to support the whole length of the chest, are laid on the x-ray table. The child lies on these, affected side *down*. A cassette is supported vertically behind the chest: the projection may either be AP or PA. The arms are raised above the head, and the knees bent (Fig. 26).

Air in the pleural cavity: the same procedure is followed, without the foam pads and with the affected side *up*.

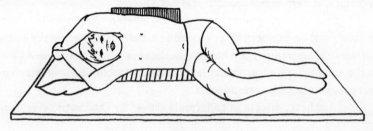

Fig. 26.

Diaphragm movement

A sub-phrenic abscess may occur after an appendicectomy. AP views of the diaphragm area, taken on inspiration and expiration, are helpful in diagnosis of this condition. The radiologist may wish to examine the child under fluoroscopy also.

Heart disease

Congenital heart disease is unfortunately common. It results from a variety of anatomical abnormalities, singly or in combination. The infant mortality rate from this cause used to be very high. Recent advances in surgery and anaesthesia mean that many babies can now be saved.

Cyanosis and/or heart failure indicate congenital heart disease in very young infants. Meticulously accurate positioning and full inspiration are essential in radiographs. Technique should be standardized in each x-ray department for all heart cases. As progressive liver enlargement is one of the main signs of heart failure, some radiologists require the upper abdomen to be included on a chest film. Centring is not altered; the light beam diaphragm is opened wider.

Babies with severe heart disease will be referred to a specialized centre for cardiac catheterization and angiography, to determine whether the condition is operable. Surgery may be undertaken straight-away.

Mild congenital heart disease may not be diagnosed till 1 or 2 years of age, or even later. A small defect may not be discovered till adulthood. The need for cardiac catheterization, angiography or surgery at any age is determined by the severity of the disease. In general, surgery, if necessary, is performed about 2 years of age.

Children with congenital heart disease, whether diagnosed in infancy or later, will be periodically reviewed at a heart clinic, generally in the out-patient department of a hospital in the area where they live. As well as the standard PA chest radiograph, lateral or oblique views may also be requested at these attendances.

Acquired heart disease in children is caused by rheumatic fever, now quite rare.

Ribs

Fractures of the ribs are not common in children because the rib-cage is so elastic. However, healing fractures may occasionally be found on a baby's chest radiograph taken for a quite unrelated reason and may be the first indication of otherwise unsuspected non-accidental injury (battered-baby syndrome).

Hydrocephalus with shunt

The request for x-ray examination of the chest (and probably skull) in a hydrocephalic child with a malfunctioning shunt needs further expla-nation. See Chapter 13 page 153.

CHAPTER 3
THE SKULL

One of the commonest requests in accident and emergency departments is for skull radiographs of head injuries. These range from a mild bump on the head in seemingly quite unaffected toddlers to severe injuries caused by road accidents or falls from a height. The routine varies in different hospitals: some admit all head injuries for twenty-four hours; some admit only those which have resulted in a period of unconsciousness or show other clinical signs, or those which prove on x-ray examination to have a fracture. In some hospitals all bumps on the head are x-rayed, no matter how slight, mainly for medico-legal reasons. This often seems a waste of time and effort to a hard-pressed radiographer dealing with a resistant toddler. However, if the policy of your hospital is to x-ray them all, then you must try to produce at least adequate AP and lateral views.

GENERAL POINTS

(1) *Do not use headclamps*: to be at all effective they have to be unacceptably tight and will upset and frighten the child.

(2) Unless the films are taken erect (when it may be found more convenient) a PA projection is not essential. Even on older children the AP projection is quite satisfactory. The lateral view can also be done with the patient supine. Children's necks are so flexible that if a child turns his head on one side, with a 45° foam pad placed under the opposite shoulder, his head will lie naturally in an almost perfect lateral position.

(3) Requests for skull examination in a ward with the mobile machine should be discussed with the doctor concerned. It is rarely possible to produce good enough films. Almost always the patient can be brought

to the department, or the examination deferred until he is fit enough for this.

(4) From the point of view of exposures, a child's head is fully grown by 5–6 years but the bone structure is not quite as dense as an adult's.

(5) Use short exposure times: 0·08–0·06 s for older children and 0·04 s for toddlers. Adjust other factors accordingly.

HEAD INJURIES

Mild injuries

AP and lateral views usually suffice; a Towne's view also if the bump was on the back of the head.

Older children

The skull unit, if available, should be used for children over about 8 years of age and the films taken in the erect position.

Small children

Co-operative children between 3 and 7 years old will find it easier to keep still lying on the x-ray table. Also, a shorter exposure time is possible if the overcouch tube is used instead of the skull unit. Reluctant 3–4 year olds are dealt with as though they were younger.

Babies and toddlers

As always when dealing with the under 3 years age-group, *get everything ready first* before you put the child on the table: cassette in Bucky tray, tube centred, field size adjusted, exposure set, compression band ready, 45° foam pad on either side of where the head will lie, a lead coat on parent or nurse. If a Towne's view is to be taken, ask mother to open buttons, zip or other fasteners on the back of the child's dress or jersey. They can then be removed to each side when the child is lying down.

Some people recommend wrapping small children tightly in a sheet to pinion their arms to their sides for radiography of the skull. Personally, I feel that this is helpful only with an infant under 3 or 4 months (Fig. 27). Once a baby is old enough to take an interest in his surroundings, the less he is restricted the better. The more you tie him up, the more likely he is to struggle and get upset. If he wants to suck his thumb,

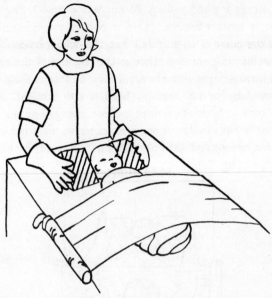

Fig. 27.

let him; or if he has a dummy this may quieten him better than any restriction. Neither will interfere with your positioning or obscure anything relevant.

AP view
Ask the mother to lay the child on the table with his head in the square of light from the light beam diaphragm. Talk to him if his mother does not. Tell him to watch the light and say when it goes out. If he lies still do not restrain him; just show mother how to hold his head straight with foam blocks while explaining to him what she is doing. Do not cover his ears (Fig. 28).

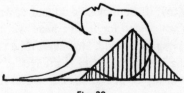

Fig. 28.

If he is struggling and yelling, do not waste time trying to distract him: speed is more effective. (This is one of the occasions when a second radiographer is invaluable.) Put the compression band, fairly tight, across his hips; stand mother at the top end of the table, firmly holding his head straight with the foam pads. Expose at the end of a yell, watching carefully to see that his head is still straight. If he keeps arching his back to look upwards at mother, change her position to the side of the table. She should put one arm across his chest and keep talking to him so that he looks down at her. She can still steady his head straight in this position (Fig. 29).

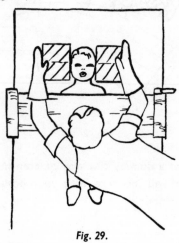

Fig. 29.

Towne's view
The Towne's view is taken in the same way. Repositioning of the head if necessary, is done *last*.

Lateral view
Put a 45° foam block under one shoulder, turn his head to the other side. Get mother to catch his attention at *the level of the table edge* with a rattle or a squeaky toy. If she moves it up and down so that it appears and disappears, he will watch for it. His head will lie in a true lateral position without having to be held. However, if he cannot be distracted and is struggling, the best immobilizer is a length of flannel orthopaedic bandage held very firmly as in Fig. 30. Do not cover his eyes with it. Tighten the compression band across his hips first.

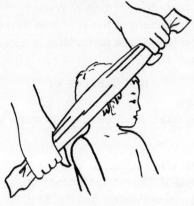

Fig. 30.

Infants

Under 3–4 months an infant's skull is not often x-rayed for suspected fracture, but may be for unusual shape, or sudden increase in size, or because of convulsions.

Try to arrange the examination for just after a feed. Often then the infant will sleep peacefully and you will have no trouble in positioning and immobilization. If this cannot be arranged, he should have something to suck while the films are being taken. Mothers can usually provide a bottle or a dummy if asked.

Before you lay him down in position, rewrap the blanket or shawl so that it comes no higher than shoulder level: folds behind the neck may appear on the Towne's view. A sandbag each side of the infant's body will hold him securely in place. For the lateral view, turn the whole baby on his side (the head and shoulders are much the same width at this age) and replace the sandbags as before. Wait a few moments for him to settle down again before taking the film.

Severe head injuries

If a head injury is caused by a road accident or fall from a height, the child may have other injuries also. Adapt your technique to take all films without moving the patient, i.e. supine on the stretcher (as with adult casualties).

The lateral view for children over 12 years should be taken with a horizontal beam if a fracture of the skull base is suspected. This will show a possible fluid level in the sphenoids.

Additional views

Depressed fracture
A tangential view is taken, localized to the injured area.

Facial bones
Injury to the facial bones requires an occipito-mental view, with base line at 45° to the vertical. This is taken as an AP projection when dealing with stretcher patients or toddlers (see Fig. 32 p. 50).

Orbit rim
(i)   Lateral view, as for paranasal sinuses.
(ii) Occipito-mental view, undertilted by 10°.

Nasal bones
(i)   Lateral view centred on nasion.
(ii) Occipito-mental view, as for antra.

(X-ray examination of the nose may also be requested for presence of a foreign body, as a small child will sometimes stuff things up his nose just to see what happens.)

Mandible
Fractures of the mandible are unusual in children. PA and lateral oblique views are taken, as in adults.

BABY'S MANDIBLE

Sometimes x-ray examination is requested to elucidate the cause of a swelling of a baby's jaw (abscess, osteomyelitis, etc.).

A *lateral oblique* is the most useful view. The baby lies supine, immobilized as for lateral view of the skull, with a cassette in position under the side of the face. The tube is angled 10°–15° towards the head, the central ray passing between the rami. The exact angulation depends on the size of the baby and the size of the swelling. The x-ray field is localized to the area of the baby's jaw.

THE PITUITARY FOSSA

The pituitary fossa is x-rayed in cases of growth abnormalities. One lateral view of the whole skull is usually preferred to a coned view of the sella turcica. Check with the radiologist which he prefers.

THE MASTOIDS

Mastoiditis in children is quite common. A toddler with acute mastoiditis will be very fractious and difficult, needing patient and sympathetic handling. An older child with a chronic, rather than acute, condition will probably co-operate well enough for a submento-vertex view to be taken if considered useful. If a skull unit is available, and the child co-operative, all views should be taken with it. A small child with an acute infection should be x-rayed supine with the overcouch tube.

Routine views
'Slit' Towne's view
The same as for an adult: the patient can be supine or erect depending on age and ability to keep still.

Lateral oblique view
Both sides are always taken for comparison. The head is in the true lateral position; the x-ray field is limited to give a coned view of the mastoid air cells; the tube is angled 20° to the feet. If the skull unit is not being used, centring must be done from the opposite (i.e. uppermost) side. Centre the cross-lines of the light beam diaphragm as in Fig. 31.

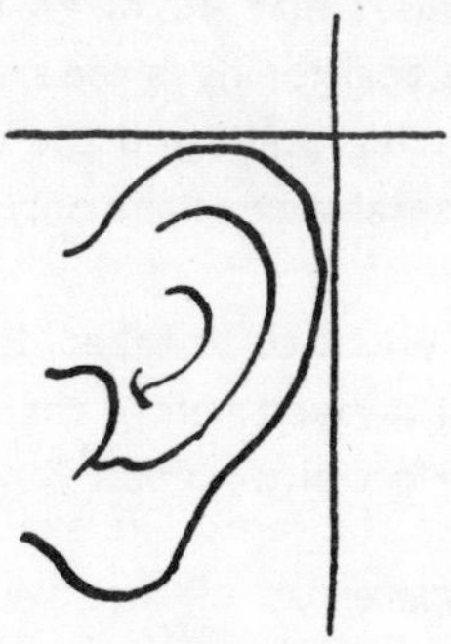

Fig. 31.

‹Slit ' submento-vertex view

Place a chair sideways in front of the skull unit, or upright Bucky. The
child sits facing the tube, holding the chair-back with one hand. He
leans back to put the crown of his head against the cassette. Children's
necks are so flexible, by comparison with adults, that this position causes
no difficulty. Demonstrate the position to the child, it is easier than
explaining. Close the light beam diaphragm to give a slit view of the
petrous bone and mastoid area. A 5° tilt of the tube upwards may be
necessary to clear the mandible from the mastoid region.

THE PARANASAL SINUSES

Requests for x-ray examination of the sinuses in children are frequent
in general hospitals which have a paediatric ear, nose and throat department. It is usually considered sufficient to take one occipito-mental
projection, as the frontal sinuses are not visible until after about 6 years
of age. An occipito-frontal projection is of little value and is rarely
required. The post-nasal space, for adenoid enlargement, is demonstrated
on a lateral projection.

These films are most easily taken in the erect position; the child is
steadier sitting rather than standing. Use the adult chest stand, he can
then hold on to the cassette holder. A stationary grid is unnecessary if a
long sinus cone is available. He should sit on a chair rather than a stool.
It is then easier for you to move him closer to the film if necessary.

Routine views

A lateral view of the sinuses may be taken routinely as well as the
occipito-mental view. The positioning is the same as for the view of the
post-nasal space; the centring point and the extent of the x-ray field
are slightly different. A lateral view is the only one taken if the request
is for the post-nasal space.

Start with this view if one is to be taken. It is more reassuring for a
child who has never been x-rayed before than if you start (as is usual
with adults) by taking the occipito-mental view.

Lateral view of post-nasal space

Seat the child facing a 13 × 18 cm (6 × 4 in) cassette. Tell him to turn his head to one side. If he is looking to the left, he should hold the cassette holder with his left hand only, the other should grip the chair seat. It helps him to keep still if there is a picture or transfer on the wall at the level of his eyes. Explain that you want him to breathe in slowly through his nose, with mouth shut, when you take the picture. This ensures that the post-nasal space is full of air, against which enlarged adenoids are clearly seen. Adjust the head to a true lateral position. Use a long sinus cone. Centre to the ramus of the mandible.

Lateral view of sinuses
Positioning is the same. The cassette can be a size larger (18 × 24 cm, 8 × 6 in). Extend the x-ray field to include all the sinuses. Centre to the outer canthus of the eye, as for adults.

Occipito-mental view
The child holds the chest stand with both hands and puts his chin on the cassette. Adjust his head position so that it is quite straight and his nose is just touching the cassette. It is very easy to overtilt for this projection as children's necks are so flexible. (The resulting film will appear to be full of teeth!)

If an *occipito-frontal view* is required, proceed as for an adult patient.

Babies and toddlers
Opinions vary among radiologists as to the usefulness of sinus radiographs of children under 3 years of age. It is thought by many that difficulty of interpretation can cause misleading results and that it is better not to take them at all. The post-nasal space view is a different matter and may be necessary at any age.

Occipito-mental view (supine)
If you have to take a sinus view of a child under 3 years it is easier to do this with the child supine. The positioning is the same as for an AP skull view, except that a 35° foam wedge is placed under the shoulders, thick end under the neck (Fig. 32). The compression band is tightened across the child's chest; tuck his arms under it if this does not upset him too much. Mother stands at the head end of the table and keeps his head straight with foam blocks. Put the cone on the x-ray tube *before* you put the child on the table.

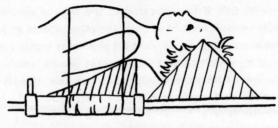

Fig. 32.

Post-nasal space view

The post-nasal space view of a resistant toddler is best done in the same way as a lateral view of the skull (see p. 44), using of course a small field, a small film, and no Potter–Bucky.

If you have a means of sitting a small child sideways in front of a chest stand which will hold a 13 × 18 cm (8 × 6 in) film at the correct height, it is sometimes possible to take a lateral post-nasal space view erect, even with babies providing they can sit up unsupported. Centre the tube and film at an appropriate height first, then put baby sitting so that his shoulders and hips are at right angles to the cassette. Mother stands in front of him and holds his hands on his thighs (Fig. 33). If he is not upset, and she can distract his attention and keep him looking at her, by watching carefully you can 'snap' a film without other immobilization.

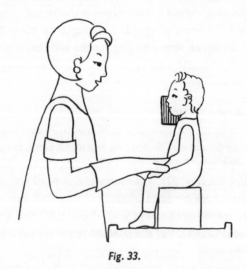

Fig. 33.

It is surprising how often this technique can produce a true lateral projection. It can also be used for a lateral view of the neck in babies with, for instance, croup. An 18 × 24 cm (8 × 6 in) film is used and the child's shoulder, not his cheek, is against the cassette.

A very short exposure time is essential in either case. It should be no longer than 0·03 s, less if possible.

CHAPTER 4
GENERAL REMARKS ON LIMB BONES

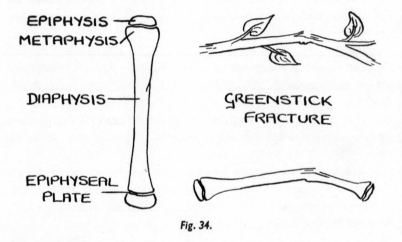

Fig. 34.

Diaphysis—shaft
Metaphysis—part of the shaft next to the epiphyseal plate
Epiphyses—ossification centre at the end of the shaft
Epiphyseal plate—cartilage layer between metaphysis and epiphysis, not visible on a radiograph.

(1) Fractures may be greenstick or complete. The younger the child, the more likely it is to be a greenstick fracture. It is similar to the result of bending a green twig to snapping point. The cortex cracks on one side and buckles on the other.

(2) The injuries that in adults produce a complete break of a long bone, in children often result in greenstick fractures or slipped epiphyses.

(3) In fractures of the long bones in children, overlap remoulds to a remarkable extent. The fractured bone grows faster and will overcome shortening of up to 1 inch or so, to equal the length of the uninjured limb.

(4) Osteomyelitis is an infective condition of bone, which may be acute or chronic. Common sites are:

upper end of tibia	upper end of femur
lower end of femur	upper end of humerus

The acute infection is extremely painful. Movement causes great distress. However, radiologically bone destruction does not show for 10–14 days. So if your radiographs show apparently normal bones, do not assume the child is making a fuss about nothing and treat him impatiently. If he *has* got osteomyelitis, even gentler handling than usual is required.

(5) Soft tissues should always be shown on orthopaedic films. They should not be blacked out by exposure factors chosen to give optimum contrast.

(6) It is useful to note exposure factors on the index card of patients who will have several follow-up films, especially when this will be to show destruction and regeneration of bone.

(7) It is not necessary to take extra views of bone abnormalities which may appear on routine views taken of a patient coming through the casualty department. He will be referred to the orthopaedic surgeon who will request other views he considers useful.

(8) For diagnosis of an injury, x-ray examination of both joints for comparison may be requested. X-ray the injured joint first, and show the film to the casualty officer. If it is still considered necessary, x-ray the other joint. Doctors who are not used to looking at paediatric radiographs often find difficulty with the many ossification centres, especially at the elbow.

(9) After diagnosis, radiography should be kept to a minimum. In post-reduction fractures and dislocations, good bone detail is not necessary. So if you have misjudged exposure factors (thickness of plaster, etc.), show the film to the surgeon or radiologist; you may be able to avoid repeating it. Even if under- or overexposed, it may provide all the information that is needed.

(10)   As a general rule, allow a child to move his own injured limb into the position you require. Most will co-operate readily, considering it preferable to the possibility of being hurt if you position it. First explain, and demonstrate, exactly the position you want. Even if he says it is impossible, a little patience and encouragement will achieve it eventually. Never try to bully a child into adopting a painful position. You will only cause fear and resentment, and a lot of trouble for the radiographer who deals with him next time.

(11)   Include the whole length of each bone with both joints on the initial film for suspected fracture, as it may be oblique or spiral.

(12)   Plaster on children's limbs is thinner than on adults. You need less increase in kilovoltage than you might think. (It is impossible to give exposure factors, as different speed screens are customarily used for plaster radiographs.)

(13)   Multiple injuries caused by road accidents or falls from a height may include trauma to abdominal and chest organs, as well as bony injuries. As with adults, adapt your technique to achieve AP and lateral projections without moving the patient. In horizontal beam techniques, be careful to cone inside the cassette edges. The primary beam should not be aimed at the body behind, e.g. an arm.

(14)   Foreign bodies: the limb should not be moved into the lateral position. Use a horizontal beam at right angles to the AP beam.

(15)   It is difficult to demonstrate the femoral head through plaster in the age group 6–18 months. Tomography is sometimes suggested. For each film of a tomographic series, the radiation dose is roughly double that of a 'plain' film. The patient is 5 times more likely to be a little girl than a boy. It is almost impossible to protect the ovaries with complete accuracy in a plaster spica. So, a high kilovoltage technique with the finest focal spot available, or a single 10° angle zonogram, is preferable, by far. The level of the zonogram 'cut' must be very accurately calculated to avoid a repeat film (see also pp. 72, 75).

CHAPTER 5
THE SHOULDER JOINT AND UPPER LIMB

THE SHOULDER

Children's shoulders are x-rayed for injuries, but not for degenerative conditions as is commonly the case with adults.

Dislocation

Dislocation is rare before adolescence, when it may be caused by a fall on the football field, or when horse riding. A single AP radiograph should be sufficient to demonstrate the injury; only if it does not provide conclusive evidence need a lateral view be taken.

AP view
The easiest way to take this is to seat the patient in front of the chest stand. Whether or not a stationary grid is used depends on the youngster's muscular development, and the amount of soft tissue swelling present. This projection alone will almost always show the presence of an *anterior* dislocation.

Lateral view
Very rarely, an additional view may be considered essential to rule out the extremely rare *posterior* dislocation. A second view of the shoulder joint ideally should be the axial projection. In practice, a patient with an injured shoulder probably will not abduct his arm enough for this. A carefully-positioned true lateral view of the scapula may serve instead.

The child sits or stands sideways to the cassette with the injured arm hanging by his side, the shoulder touching the cassette. He is then rotated forwards towards the cassette until the plane of the scapula is at right angles to it. The x-ray field is limited to the area of scapula and upper third of humerus. This should provide a 'skyline' view of a posteriorly dislocated humeral head.

THE CLAVICLE

Fracture

Fracture of the clavicle is very common in children of all ages, usually in mid-shaft. Lying down is painful, so take the radiograph in the erect position, unless your patient is a baby or a stretcher case.

AP view
Put a cassette, large enough to include the whole length of the clavicle, crosswise in the chest stand. Seat the child in front of it, facing the x-ray tube. (Teenagers can be positioned PA as for adults.) Adjust his position so that the clavicle is approximately parallel to the film. If he is old enough to hold his breath explain you will want him to do so; if not, use a very short exposure time (0·02 s). Limit the x-ray field to the clavicle.

Infero-superior view
If no fracture is demonstrated on the AP view, repeat with a 10°–15° tilt upwards of the x-ray tube, to project the clavicle above the ribs.

Birth injuries in the new born
The commonest sites for fractures caused by a difficult delivery are the clavicle and humerus. One AP projection, with the infant supine, to confirm a fracture of the bone in question, is sufficient.

THE HUMERUS

Fractures

Fractures of the humerus are less common than in adults. They can occur anywhere along the shaft. As with a fractured clavicle, it is less painful for the child if you seat or stand him in front of the chest stand and take the films erect rather than supine.

AP view

Use a film large enough to include the whole shaft of the bone. You will probably find you need a 30 × 40 cm (15 × 12 in) cassette. Though it may seem wasteful, use another the same size for the lateral view. Make sure the head of the humerus is not going to be obscured by the patient's name. If your department has a lead-rubber apron for chest radiography, fasten it as in Fig. 35 to protect the body from scatter.

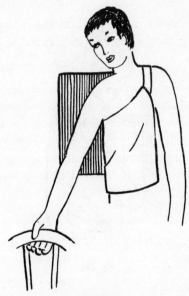

Fig. 35.

The child leans towards the injured side to abduct the arm slightly. If you can find something (such as a chair back) at the right height for him to grasp, it will help to steady him. If he can hold his breath, it will also help.

Lateral view

An adequate lateral view is obtained simply by internally rotating the arm from the AP position. Ask the child to do this himself and tell him to stop if it hurts. It is often quite easily and painlessly done, even when there is a fracture, and will not do any further damage. A small child can tuck his thumb into his trouser belt.

Post-reduction films
The treatment is immobilization of the arm in a collar-and-cuff sling, usually with a plaster U-slab. Follow-up radiographs in true AP and lateral positions will be more difficult to achieve. A little ingenuity in rotating the child and angling the x-ray tube should produce an AP view of the fracture site (Fig. 36).

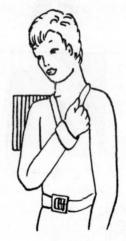

Fig. 36.

For the *lateral view*, put a cassette between the arm and chest, as high up into the axilla as possible. A nurse, or the patient with his other hand, will have to support the bottom edge of the cassette to keep it in position. You will not get the full length of the humerus on this film but you should demonstrate the fracture position adequately. If the fracture is too near the humeral head for this method, take a coned trans-thoracic projection at 6-ft distance with a lateral chest exposure.

Never remove a collar-and-cuff sling. It maintains the fracture in reduction.

Diseases

Acute osteomyelitis

The upper end of the humerus is a common site in the arm for osteo-myelitis. This acute infection is extremely painful. Try to get the child to move the arm into position himself. Handling and movement should be kept to a minimum. Take AP and lateral views as for fracture in the same place. It is helpful to show the soft tissues, as bone changes are not evident for 10–14 days.

Osteogenic sarcoma

Sarcoma is fortunately rare, usually occurring at the same site as osteomyelitis. It presents as a painful swelling at the upper end of the arm. Treat very gently, and take AP and lateral views as described above.

Bone cyst

The shaft of a cylindrical bone (usually humerus or femur) is the site of the solitary bone cyst which occurs in childhood, mostly in boys. Beginning in the metaphysis, it grows in size slowly and painlessly. The defect in the bone is filled with fluid contained within a thin membrane. Eventually a fracture is likely at the site, which is often how the presence of a bone cyst is first discovered.

The treatment is surgical. The fluid is drained and the walls of the cavity curetted. The space is filled with bone chips round which the lesion heals and solidifies into normal bone.

THE ELBOW JOINT

Injuries

When dealing with a child's injured elbow, it is not only cruel and unnecessary but may be positively dangerous to force the joint into full extension in order to obtain a true AP projection. If the injury is slight, he may do it without difficulty. If a fracture or dislocation is present, it is impossible without causing great pain and risking further damage.

Because there are several ossification centres at the elbow joint, an injury can result in a number of different fractures and/or avulsions of an epiphysis. Dislocations are not common.

Sometimes a request is made to x-ray the other elbow for comparison.

Lateral view

Start with the lateral view. A child needs a great deal of persuasion
to abduct an injured arm in order to put it on the x-ray table. Have him
stand sideways to it, injured side to the table. Be patient: explain what
you want him to do. If the arm is in a triangular sling, leave it on. You
can undo the knot and open it out when his arm is supported on the
table. He will probably be clutching the injured forearm with his good
hand. Support the upper arm on the inside with one hand, put your
other hand gently under the elbow joint, and ease it slowly over the
edge of the table. Mother or nurse puts a chair immediately behind him
and as he sits down the arm rests on the table. A small child will need
a pillow or large foam pad on the chair to bring him to the right height.
A tall child may have to slide his bottom forward on the chair seat to
bring his upper arm on the table top. You will have to judge this before
he sits down.

If your department has an upright Bucky which can be turned into
the horizontal plane, or a skull table, it is much easier. You can then
adjust the table height to bring his elbow into line with his shoulder,
rather than adjusting the child to bring his shoulder into line with his
elbow. It may not be possible to persuade him to turn his forearm into
a true lateral position. If it hurts him to do this, do not insist; he will
only raise his shoulder and you still will not get a true lateral elbow
position.

If the child is very young and upset, and the elbow swollen and tender,
you may not be able to position him in the way described above. An
alternative method is suggested under 'supracondylar fracture' (see
p. 62).

AP view

The child should move his own arm from the lateral position into whichever position you have decided on for the AP projection. Give him time,
plenty of encouragement, and physical support if you want him to stand
up.

(1)   The child stands beside the table. The forearm should lie flat on the
cassette, the back of the hand flat on the table. This is the best AP
projection for unspecified bony injury.

(2)   A second AP view should be taken if the first proves negative,

or if the pain is localized to the end of the humerus. The child sits, with the back of the upper arm in contact with the cassette, the forearm supported in the AP position on a foam pad.

In each case the child extends the elbow as far as possible, and leans slightly to the injured side. Centre to the elbow joint without angulation of the tube.

Supracondylar fracture of the humerus
The commonest fracture of the elbow joint, and potentially the most dangerous, is the supracondylar fracture. It occurs from 3 to 12 years, mostly between 5 and 8 years. The jagged edge of the humeral shaft may tear or compress the brachial artery or stretch the median nerve (Fig. 37).

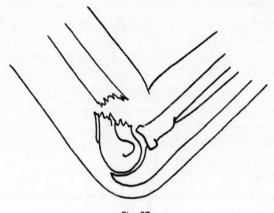

Fig. 37.

When positioning for x-ray examination there must be no movement at the joint; this can cause further damage.
(1) Do not turn the arm on the table from the lateral position into the AP position.
(2) Do not attempt to straighten the elbow joint.
(3) Use two separate cassettes for AP and lateral views.

Remember that what is needed are AP and lateral views of the lower end of the humerus; the position of the forearm bones is largely irrelevant. It is best to take both views erect, as described for the humerus.

AP view

Put a cassette in the chest stand. Seat the child sideways on a chair in front of it so that the chair-back is to his uninjured side. Have him support the forearm of the injured arm with his other hand, and remove the sling. He should lean slightly to the injured side, causing enough abduction of the arm to avoid irradiating the chest wall. Put a lead apron on, if available, as described for the humerus. Align the chair so that the upper arm contacts the cassette in the AP position (Fig. 38). Close the light beam diaphragm so that only the lower third of the humerus is in the x-ray field. If the angle of flexion is more than 90°, centre to the lower end of humerus with a horizontal beam. If the angle is less than 90°, angle the tube a little down (and displace cassette) to compensate, centring to the lower end of humerus as before.

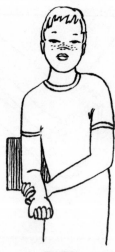

Fig. 38.

Lateral view

Prop a cassette upright on the chair seat between the elbow and the child's body, at right angles to the position of the previous AP film. Align the horizontal beam at right angles to the cassette. Centre to the lower end of the humerus. Put a piece of lead rubber behind the cassette and across his lap, to protect the gonads.

If the child arrives on a stretcher, leave the arm as it is and angle the x-ray tube to get a true AP position. Let the child lift his arm himself for you to put the film underneath. He will not make his injury worse. When he lifts his arm again for you to retrieve the film substitute a rectangular foam pad, stand the cassette upright between arm and body and use a horizontal beam to take the lateral view. Put a piece of lead rubber behind the cassette. Mother or nurse, in a lead coat, can holdthe hand of his injured arm in position.

Post-reduction films (Fig. 39)

These will be taken in theatre with the child still anaesthetized. The AP view will be taken with the arm in acute flexion, so an increase of 10 kV is necessary to penetrate the forearm.

The surgeon will lift the arm for you to put a foam pad underneath, to take a lateral view with horizontal beam; the cassette is placed between the elbow and body. As with all supine patients use lead rubber to protect the body from radiation.

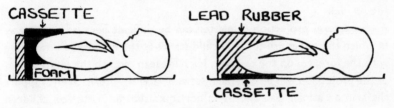

Fig. 39.

Follow-up films

This fracture is usually treated after reduction by immobilization in a collar-and-cuff sling, with elbow flexed at 20°–30° above right angles, with or without a plaster backslab.

Never remove a collar-and-cuff sling

For the early follow-up films, use the technique described above with the patient sitting on a chair and cassettes in the chest stand. The arm may be swollen and sore; treat it gently. The AP view will need an increase of 15 kV to penetrate the forearm also. Use fast screens; good bone detail is not wanted; the position of the fracture is what the surgeon needs to see. Be sure to position the lower end of the humerus in the true AP position. The radius and ulna are not important.

For later follow-up films, when the arm has ceased to hurt and the swelling subsided, the child may be able to lift his elbow on to a foam pad at the end of the table for the lateral projection. Remember to put a piece of lead rubber over his lap. The AP view is taken as for the post-reduction film.

THE FOREARM

For all projections of the forearm (and of the wrist and hand) patients should sit *sideways* to the x-ray table to remove the gonads from the primary beam.

Greenstick fractures of the radius and ulna are very common.

AP view
The first examination, which includes the full length of both bones and the elbow and wrist joints, should be in the AP position. Post-reduction films in plaster can be taken in the PA position.

Lateral view
A true lateral projection in plaster can be difficult because of the way in which the bones are set. The child stands at the end of the x-ray table with the forearm on the cassette. He must lean over to the injured side, or the projection will be oblique instead of lateral. Alternatively, support the arm on a foam pad and use a horizontal beam. Plaster on children is often much thinner than on adults and may need only an increase of as little as 5 kV. Sometimes it is only a back-slab.

Baby's arm and forearm
Sometimes a baby is taken to the accident department because he has suddenly ceased to move one arm, though there may be no history of an injury. It is convenient to x-ray the whole arm on one film.

AP view
Ask the mother to lay baby on the x-ray table. Put the compression band across his hips, with a foam pad underneath it. The top border of the cassette under the arm should be an inch or two above the shoulder. Make sure the name-space is not under the head of the humerus. Gently extend the arm flat in the AP position. Mother holds the opposite

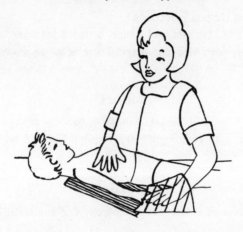

Fig. 40.

shoulder down on the table with one hand, and the hand of the injured arm, palm up, on the cassette with her other hand (Fig. 40). Protect her hand with a lead cut-out (Fig. 5 p. 7). The cutaway bit should be over the baby's wrist, so that the epiphysis is not covered. If it is possible to do so, it is a good idea to include the clavicle on this film.

If an attempt to extend the elbow joint obviously causes pain, support the forearm on a 15° or 30° foam wedge. Mother can still hold baby's hand to keep the whole arm in a true AP position.

Lateral view
Abduct the arm gently, bend the elbow and internally rotate the arm to bring elbow and forearm into the lateral position. Slide a cassette under the arm making sure the shoulder joint is on it. Mother holds as before, baby's hand being in the lateral position with the thumb upwards.

THE WRIST JOINT

Injuries
Slipped radial epiphysis
Slipped radial epiphysis is similar to an adult Colles' fracture, and is caused by the same kind of fall. Take AP and lateral views. This injury is seen usually in school-age children.

Scaphoid and carpus fractures

Fractures of the scaphoid and other carpal bones are uncommon in children, rarely seen before teenage. Treat as for an adult.

Rickets

Usually one PA wrist film is taken initially, to show changes in epiphyses and diaphyses. The radiologist may require films of other areas also (knees or rib ends).

Lead poisoning

Lead lines appear in wrists. A PA projection of one wrist is taken.

Bone age

'Bone age' means the age at which the ossification centres appear. Any deviation from the normal is most easily assessed at the wrist joint. Such information is helpful in the investigation of a child who is failing to thrive, from whatever cause, and in certain other conditions.

One PA film of wrist and hand (left or right routinely) is taken. Sometimes a radiologist may specify other centres also for more accurate assessment (foot, knee, etc.).

Radiographic techniques for the hand and wrist of small children are described in the next section.

THE HAND AND FINGERS

For injuries to the hands and fingers of older children, the technique is the same as for an adult.

Toddlers

A common injury is a toddler's hand caught in a door. Seat him on mother's knee at the edge of the x-ray table. Use separate cassettes for the *PA and oblique views.* Ask mother to lay the injured hand flat, palm down, on the cassette and keep it there by a firm grip on the forearm. If you are quick, you may manage to take a PA view before the child decides he wants his hand back again. Repeat the procedure for an oblique view, placing a 'cushion for the sore hand' (a small triangular foam pad) on the cassette to tilt the hand into the oblique position.

A *lateral view* of the fingers can be taken in the same way, by placing the hand in the lateral position. The fingers will lie naturally separated from each other. A sore finger in particular will be stuck out straight by itself; a small foam pad may be useful to support it. A very short exposure time is essential.

A co-operative 3 year old will put the hand in position and keep it there without being held. At this age the child can stand by the x-ray table, or kneel on a chair if not tall enough.

Babies

A baby, or a resistant toddler, is best dealt with supine on the table, immobilized with the compression band. Mother then has both hands free to hold baby's hand flat and still. Each finger must be uncurled and extended. A strip of clear x-ray film keeps the fingers flat (Fig. 41) and enables you to see if one has curled up again.

Request for x-ray examination of a baby's hand and wrist is usually for bone age, rather than injury.

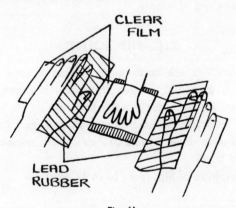

Fig. 41.

CHAPTER 6
THE PELVIS AND HIP JOINTS

THE PELVIS

Fractures

Road accidents are the cause of most fractures of the pelvis in children. The child may have intra-abdominal injuries also and will arrive on a stretcher. He must be carefully lifted on to the x-ray table on a canvas and poles by two people.

Gonad protection is important but must not obscure an injury. It is better to use none for girls on the first examination. Protection used for boys *must not* cover the pubic bones. Take one AP view of pelvis and upper third of femora.

THE HIP JOINT

Traumatic dislocations are uncommon. The adult type of fractured neck of femur is exceedingly rare. There are, however, several abnormalities which do not occur in adult patients:

(i) congenital dislocation of hip: from birth to 5 years (mostly girls);
(ii) Perthes' disease: from 4 years to 7 or 8 years, occasionally earlier or later (mostly boys);
(iii) slipped epiphysis of hip: from 10 to 17 years.

Congenital dislocation of the hip (CDH)

Congenital dislocation of the hip is an abnormality which may be secondary to conditions causing muscle imbalance or paralysis, such as myelomeningocele. But usually there is no obvious cause and the infant is otherwise normal. One or both hips may be affected.

As the success of treatment depends, to a large extent, upon the age at which it is discovered, all babies are examined at birth for hip instability. There is a special way of holding and manipulating an infant's hips to prove stability. An unstable hip is said to 'click', so 'clicking hips' may appear as a diagnosis on an x-ray form. Subluxation means a partial dislocation.

Early treatment

The newborn infant with unstable hip(s) will spend some weeks in double nappies or some form of abduction splint. Both keep the femoral head in the acetabulum as the infant grows. If a splint is used, the baby may be x-rayed in it when it is first applied.

Most authorities agree there is little to be gained from radiology for diagnosis of this condition before 12 weeks of age. Until recently, the first radiograph was an AP view of the hip joints in the Von Rosen position: 45° internal rotation and abduction. This has now been largely discarded, as it did not prove wholly accurate for assessment.

AP view of hips at 3 months

Place baby at the end of the x-ray table with a cassette under the pelvis. Mother stands at the end and holds his legs. Put the compression band,

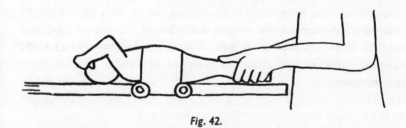

Fig. 42.

not too tightly, across his chest, to stop him trying to sit up. Don't pinion his arms under it: leave them free (Fig. 42).

The pelvis must be level, the whole length of both legs in the true AP position, knees straight, feet together, toes pointing up. Mother holds the lower legs, with her thumb or first finger on the knee joint (Fig. 43). Baby will dislike this and will resist, so warn mother to hold

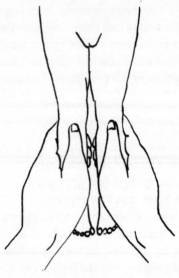

Fig. 43.

tight. A very small lead–rubber cut-out is Sellotaped to a boy's thighs or a girl's abdomen (Fig. 44).

Many babies do not need further treatment but will be reviewed again at intervals until about one year old when they commence walking. Others may have to continue in an abduction splint for a further period, during which they may be x-rayed in the splint.

Therefore, if a baby is brought to the x-ray department in a splint, enquire whether this is to be removed or left on for the x-ray examination.

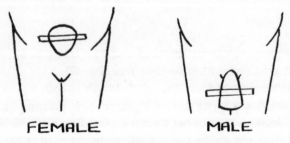

FEMALE   MALE

Fig. 44.

Later treatment

After about 6 months of age a child may be x-rayed in a variety of different traction frames (Fig. 45) or plasters plintages and during surgery. The régimes for treatment vary from one orthopaedic surgeon to another. However, the aim of all forms of treatment is the same: to reduce the dislocation and make sure it stays reduced.

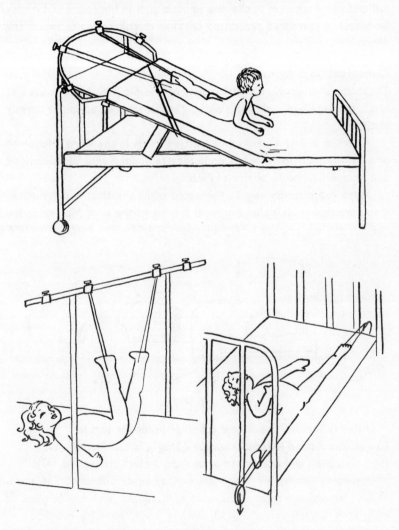

Fig. 45.

The area radiographed and the projection are the same every time, no matter at what angle to the trunk the legs may be immobilized: an AP view of the pelvis, centred just above the symphysis pubis, including the upper thirds of both femora if possible.

Every effort should be made to protect the gonads, as these children will probably have many x-ray examinations. However, it is extremely difficult to be accurate in the case of little girls in hip spicas and it may be better to leave lead protection off, than to risk having to repeat the film.

Conservative treatment

Those cases of congenital dislocation of the hip which are missed at birth, but are diagnosed before walking starts, are treated conservatively initially.

A period of 3 or 4 weeks on a traction frame in the ward is followed by an attempt at closed reduction in theatre under a general anaesthetic and immobilization in plaster of Paris.

X-ray examination may be requested while the child is on traction. If the traction is such that the child is lying prone with hips extended the film can be taken as a PA projection. A grid is not used.

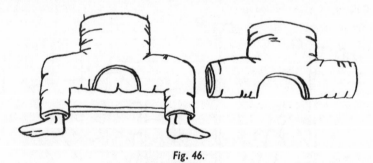

Fig. 46.

After reduction, the plaster splintage holds the legs in

(i) abduction and external rotation ('frog' plaster, Fig. 46), or
(ii) abduction and internal rotation ('Batchelor' plaster, Fig. 47).

Exposure factors for 'frog' plaster may cause difficulty. The acetabulum, femoral head and neck should be visualized. This may be possible only at a kilovoltage of 80–90, with a corresponding reduction in milliampere-seconds to 12 mAs or less. Gonad protection is 1 mm thick.

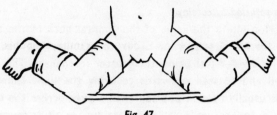

Fig. 47.

The child in a Batchelor plaster may flex the hips and cause the metal bar to obscure the hip joints. When positioning, put a sandbag over the bar to prevent this.

Surgical treatment
If conservative treatment is unsuccessful, or if the diagnosis is first made sometime after the child has started walking, surgery may be considered necessary.

(1) Open reduction
The hip is exposed, soft tissues preventing the femoral head from fitting into the acetabulum are excised, the dislocation is reduced and the pelvis and legs plastered to maintain the reduction. The hip spica will be the full length of both legs, with the affected leg in abduction and internal rotation (Fig. 48).

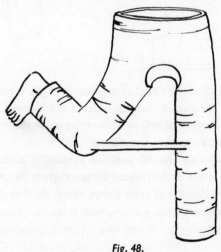

Fig. 48.

(2) *Varus rotation osteotomy*

This operation alters the angle of the femoral neck to the shaft. It is often considered necessary in order to stabilize the reduced hip. The femur is divided just below the greater trochanter. The distal part is adducted and rotated outwards to bring the knee facing straight ahead. It is usually held in position with a plate across the osteotomy site. Some surgeons use a nail-and-plate (as for adult fractured neck of femur). Radiography may be needed during this operation.

A plaster hip spica enclosing the pelvis and one or both legs (Fig. 49) may be applied after the osteotomy and removed some weeks later.

Sometimes open reduction and osteotomy are performed at the same operation.

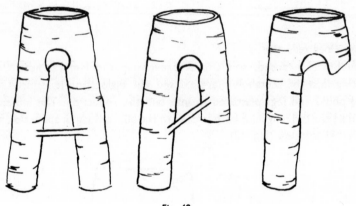

Fig. 49.

Follow-up films should include the whole length of the plate and all the screws, whichever method of internal fixation is employed. An *AP view* is sufficient while the child is still in a plaster spica. A *lateral view* is also taken, once the plaster has been removed.

Rotate the child from the AP position 45° to the side in question. Both knee and hip joints of the treated leg are slightly flexed. The other knee is bent also until the foot rests flat on the table. The knees should be wide apart. Centre to the groin crease (Fig. 50). Place the gonad protection very carefully, so as not to obscure any part of the hip or femur.

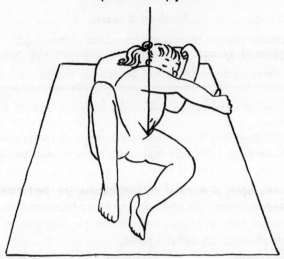

Fig. 50.

(3) Acetabular reconstruction

Dislocation undetected before the child has started to walk, or those cases which pose particular difficulties in management, may be considered to require surgery to reconstruct the acetabulum. A common procedure is called 'Salter's pelvic osteotomy' (Fig. 51). A piece of bone is taken from the ilium and inserted to form an extension to the acetabular roof.

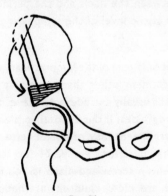

Fig. 51.

All radiographs taken of the hips in a plaster spica after surgery need a grid and a kilovoltage of 90–100 kV, with 8–10 mAs. Use 1 mm thick· gonad protection.

Perthes' disease

Perthes' disease consists of an avascular necrosis of the femoral epiphysis
and may be bilateral. The cause is unknown. It can be painless or there
may be referred pain in the knee. Sometimes the only symptom is a
limp.

On the initial examination, two views are taken of both hips.

AP view

The pelvis must be level, the legs quite straight with the knee caps
aligned symmetrically in the true AP position. The feet are together,
with the toes pointing upwards. A sandbag against the outside of each
ankle helps to maintain the position. The lead protection should not lie
over the pubic rami in a boy, nor obscure the acetabulum in a girl.
Centre just above the symphysis pubis.

Frog lateral view

The knees are flexed and separated as widely as possible. The soles of
the feet are brought together. It may not be possible to abduct the
affected hip joint as far as the good one and this will cause the pelvis
to tilt. So adjust the legs at equal angles to the pelvis. Because in this
position there is no support for the lead protection on a boy, it is easy
to make the mistake of placing it too high over the pubis. To avoid this,
use a foam block between the heels and the perineum, to support the
piece of lead rubber at the level of the symphysis pubis (Fig. 52).

Treatment

If the damage involves only part of the femoral head, without subluxation,
there may be no treatment other than review at intervals. Follow-up
x-ray examination will usually include both views of both hips.

As the disease progresses, if the femoral epiphysis shows a tendency
to subluxation, the treatment may require a varus rotation osteotomy,
rather similar to that described on p. 74 for congenital dislocation
of the hip. A Coventry screw-and-plate is commonly used for this
osteotomy, as these are older children in whom the weight-bearing
load is proportionately greater. X-ray control may be needed for the
operation.

A post-operative film is usually taken before the child leaves the
theatre. A grid is necessary only if a plaster hip spica has been applied·

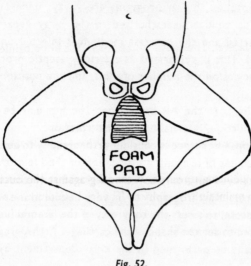

Fig. 52.

After discharge from hospital the child will attend the out-patient clinic at intervals for a year or so. *Follow-up films* taken during this time should always show the full length of the plate and all the screws. It is usual to take an AP view of both hips and either a frog lateral of both or a lateral (as described on p. 74) of just the plated hip.

About a year later, the Coventry screw-and-plate is removed.

Some orthopaedic surgeons consider a Salter's osteotomy to be preferable to a varus osteotomy in certain cases.

Arthrography

If difficulty is experienced in obtaining closed reduction of a dislocated hip due to obstructing soft tissues, some orthopaedic surgeons consider an arthrogram helpful. Most often this is done in theatre, when the child has already been anaesthetized prior to an attempt at manipulative reduction.

The surgeon inserts a lumbar puncture needle through the joint capsule, under fluoroscopic control if mobile screening equipment is available. Two to three millilitres of Hypaque 25% (or similar) is injected and the needle is withdrawn. The number of films taken and the position of the hip joint, is decided by the surgeon.

In some hospitals, hip arthrograms are always undertaken by the radiologist. The child is anaesthetized in the x-ray department. The needle is inserted and the contrast medium is injected under fluoroscopic control. This is performed as a strictly aseptic procedure. The radiologist decides on the number of films, and the positions of the hip joint.

Radiography is in the AP projection. The hip may be in neutral, adduction, abduction, internal or external rotation.

Some orthopaedic surgeons consider arthrography to be unnecessary in the management of congenital dislocation of the hip as the joint will have to be explored surgically anyhow, if closed reduction is unobtainable. Some consider arthrography to be very helpful in the management of Perthes' disease, to assess the congruity of the femoral head with the acetabulum, and to see the shape of the cartilage. Arthrography of these cases will usually be performed in the x-ray department by the radiologist.

Slipped upper femoral epiphysis

A less common condition than the previous two, slipped upper femoral epiphysis is likely to occur in (usually overweight) teenage children. It is due to hormonal imbalance and may be precipitated by an injury. Often the slip, which is backwards and downwards, is visible only on the lateral film.

An *AP view* of both hips is taken at the first examination.

As the break in continuity is between the femoral neck and head, there is a similarity to an adult fractured neck of femur.

The correct *lateral view* therefore is as for the adult fracture: a true lateral of the femoral neck, using a horizontal beam with the patient supine.

Treatment

The femoral epiphysis is usually stabilized with three stainless steel pins (Fig. 53). The operative procedure is similar to the pinning of an adult fracture. *AP* and *lateral views* are taken of the inserted pin(s) as requested by the surgeon; or fluoroscopy is employed if available.

When there is no fluoroscopic unit, two mobile x-ray machines must be employed. They are set in position after the child has been anaes-

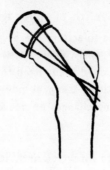

Fig. 53.

thetized and transferred to the orthopaedic table. Once aligned for the AP and lateral projections, they are not moved again till after the operation.

Exact centring and coning should be ascertained before both child and x-ray tubes disappear under theatre towels. You should also check that you can place and retrieve cassettes without interfering with the sterile drapes.

Follow-up films
Post-operatively, the patient may be on traction in bed for 2–3 weeks. After discharge he will attend the out-patient clinic at intervals for a year. He is then readmitted to hospital for removal of the pins.

During this time the unaffected hip is kept under review also. X-ray examination at out-patient attendances will usually include both hips.

Transient synovitis of hip

Also known as 'irritable hip', transient synovitis of the hip occurs from 2 to 10 years of age. The cause is unknown. There is a fairly sudden onset of pain and stiffness in the affected joint. One *AP view* of both hips is taken when the child is admitted to hospital. If this proves negative, a *frog lateral* may be requested also to exclude other conditions.

The treatment is bed-rest on traction for a week. If all symptoms have disappeared the child is discharged and attends the next out-patient clinic. He may be x-rayed again as an out-patient.

Acute osteomyelitis of upper end of femur

Osteomyelitis is a pyogenic infection, the acute form of which is extremely painful. Treat very gently. One *AP view* of both hips is taken in the department before the child is admitted to a ward.

A *lateral view* is not routinely taken, as movement causes a great deal of pain and in any case, bone changes do not show until from 10 to 14 days later.

Acute infective arthritis

The same remarks apply to this condition. It is caused either by osteomyelitis of the femur, as an abscess invading the hip joint, or by blood-borne infection from another site.

Tuberculosis

Tubercular infection of the hip joint is rare nowadays. It is not so painful as acute osteomyelitis, and it may prove possible to take a *frog lateral view*, if required, without causing too much distress.

These last three infections are all treated by bed-rest and traction for a number of weeks, or even months. Bone destruction and regeneration are assessed periodically by x-ray examination. As these films are all taken with the mobile machine on the ward, great care must be taken to ensure that they are of the highest standard possible, showing optimum bone detail. A grid should be used only if you can be absolutely sure that it is exactly at right angles to the x-ray beam. A sinus cone can be used instead, provided it covers a field big enough to include the whole of the infected area. Exposure factors should be noted on the child's card, or first set of films, and used for all follow-up radiography.

CHAPTER 7
THE LOWER LIMB

THE FEMUR

Fractures

The commonest cause of fractured femur in children is a road traffic accident. The fracture is most often in the mid-shaft. The child will arrive on a stretcher with the leg in a splint. You must try, as far as possible, to get true AP and lateral projections of the whole length of the femur, without removing the splint. The lateral view is most easily obtained with a horizontal beam, placing the cassette against the outside of the injured leg. There may be an associated dislocation of the hip. So the initial examination should include an AP view of the hip joint also. Gonad protection should be carefully placed so as not to obscure the pubic rami or acetabulum.

Post-reduction AP view

The child is admitted for treatment which consists of traction in a Thomas' splint, sometimes suspended from an overhead beam. He is x-rayed again within the next 24 h. The 'beam' is nowadays made of metal and runs the length of the bed, causing difficulty for the first post-reduction AP projection. At this time the child will be still upset and frightened from the accident. He probably will not even speak to you. Explain what you are going to do, even if he seems not to be listening. It is important to be particularly kind and gentle this first time, so that he will not mind subsequent x-ray examinations in the following weeks. Do not try to position for the AP view unaided. Get a nurse to lift him while you slide the film underneath. In doing this, ease him out gently sideways from under the traction beam, otherwise it will almost completely obscure the femur on the radiograph.

The leg will probably be in slight external rotation in the Thomas' splint: do not attempt to correct this. It is better, for the first post-reduction films, to take two radiographs at right angles of the leg as it presents in the splint. If the orthopaedic surgeon insists on exact AP and lateral projections, you will have to tilt the tube as necessary to obtain them.

Post-reduction lateral view
Support the film vertically against the outside of the thigh with a 45° foam block. Use a horizontal beam. Beware of irradiating the child in the next bed. If the fracture is in the upper third of the femur, lead gonad protection may obscure it.

After a week or so the child will happily move anywhere in the bed for his follow-up x-ray examinations.

Babies in gallows traction
Fractured femur in children under 2 years is treated by traction in a gallows frame (Fig. 54). Special difficulties are caused radiographically by the fact that both legs are suspended and that the frame is in a cot, not a bed. The cot bars must be avoided in the AP projection and the uninjured leg in the lateral. Both films are taken with a horizontal beam.

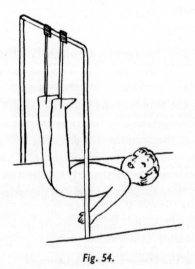

Fig. 54.

AP view

Ask Sister's permission to move the cot, and for a nurse to help. You must have enough room to get the x-ray tube with the beam directed horizontally at the head end of the cot. Support a 15 × 40 cm (15 × 6 in) cassette against the back of the leg with a 45° foam block and sandbag (Fig. 55). The light-beam-diaphragm box should be against the cot bars: the shadows of the bars can be clearly seen and must not overlie the leg.

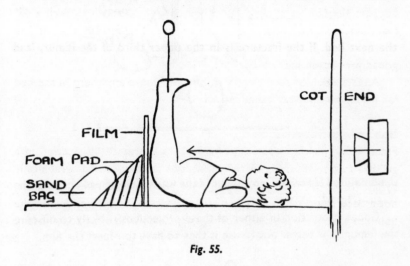

Fig. 55.

You may have to off-centre sideways a fraction to throw them clear. Cone to the outline of the thigh. Make sure no one is standing in, or about to walk past, the direct line of the x-ray beam. If the baby is very fractious and will not keep still, nurse or mother in a lead apron holds the leg and top edge of the cassette.

Lateral view

For the first post-reduction film you may not be able to separate the legs, without hurting and thoroughly upsetting baby. Support the cassette against the outside of the thigh with foam block and sandbag as before (Fig. 56). The cotside is let down, and the x-ray beam centred to the uninjured femur. You have now two thicknesses of leg to penetrate, so increase the kilovoltage by 7–10 kV. In subsequent examinations

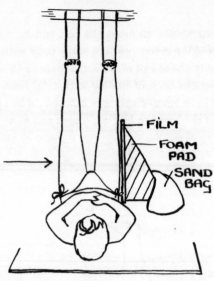

Fig. 56.

the uninjured leg can be moved out of the way by a foam pad between the thighs (Fig. 57).

Gonad protection in either of these projections is likely to obscure the femur. It is better not to use it than to have to repeat the film.

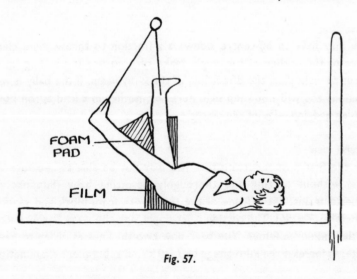

Fig. 57.

Diseases

Acute osteomyelitis

The lower end of the femur is a common site for osteomyelitis. So is the upper end of the tibia. The request form may specify the knee as the area to be examined. It is important to use large enough films, not the 18 × 24 cm (8 × 6 in) size used for the knee joint; 15 × 40 cm (15 × 6 in) will include an adequate length of femur and tibia. The knee is not flexed at right angles for the lateral view. In fact, the condition is so painful it may be necessary to take this view with a horizontal beam, the leg being raised on rectangular foam pads (Fig. 58).

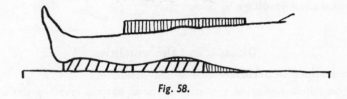

Fig. 58.

Sarcoma

The lower end of the femur is the most usual site for this rare condition also. It presents as a painful swelling. AP and lateral films are taken. Include the knee joint on the film, but centre above it, so as to demonstrate a greater length of femur than of tibia on the radiograph.

Bone cyst   see p. 59.

THE KNEE JOINT

Some radiologists prefer both knees to be included on the initial AP view with a lateral view only of the affected knee.

AP view

It is difficult to keep the knees fully extended when sitting upright on the x-ray table, or when lying supine. If the fluorescent screen carriage is normally parked across the end of the table, a pillow against this provides a convenient backrest. Otherwise the child should lean backwards supported on his elbows. A sandbag each side of the lower leg prevents rotation of the limb.

Lateral view

The child turns to the affected side, again leaning on his elbow. The uppermost leg should be quite straight. The knee in question is flexed to 45° and a foam pad placed under the ankle.

The patella

A fracture of the patella is caused by direct violence, e.g. a kick in a football game, or indirect violence when the knee is forcibly flexed. If the recommended *PA view* is not possible because of pain, take an *AP view* and double the milliampere-seconds. A *lateral view* is taken in the same way as for the knee joint, but centre over the patella and decrease the kilovoltage by 5 kv.

Diseases and abnormalities

Acute infective arthritis

Osteomyelitis may cause the infection as an abscess invading the knee joint. This and the following condition are treated by traction in bed, so the follow-up examinations will be done in the ward with the mobile machine. Beware of irradiating the child in the next bed when using a horizontal beam.

Tuberculosis

Tuberculosis of the knee is rare nowadays, and is secondary to pulmonary tuberculosis, so initially the chest is x-rayed also.

Osgood–Schlatter's disease

Osteochondritis of the tibial tubercle is called Osgood–Schlatter's disease. Lateral views should be taken of both knees. An AP view is sometimes requested also, in case the symptoms are caused by some other condition. Reduce the usual lateral exposure by 5 kV.

Osteochondritis dissecans

This affects teenagers. It can occur in other joints but is most frequently found in the knee. It is best demonstrated by a *tunnel view*. Part of the femoral articular surface and a fragment of underlying bone dies and becomes separated, either partially when it remains in place, or completely when it becomes a 'loose body' within the joint space.

Exostosis

The term exostosis includes osteoma (a benign tumour of bone tissue) and osteochondroma (the same composed of bone and cartilage tissue).

Shaped like a small spur, an exostosis grows out from (usually) the upper end of the tibia, or the lower end of the femur. A *tangential view*, with the exostosis on the 'skyline', will show its extent. It may be invisible on the usual AP and lateral views of the knee.

Knock knees

Knock knees is a postural abnormality which is not often x-rayed. If it is required, an AP film of both knees should be taken, with the child standing. Rarely, surgical correction may be needed in early teenage.

THE TIBIA AND FIBULA

Fractures

Fractures are quite common in the lower third of the tibia and may be associated with a fracture of the upper end of the fibula, so include both knee and ankle joints on initial films. Treatment, as in adults, is by immobilization of the whole leg in plaster after reduction.

Post-reduction AP view

As the knee is flexed at 5° angle in plaster, a foam pad should be placed under the knee. The tube is angled slightly to project the central ray at right angles to the tibial shaft. A sandbag against the foot prevents rotation of the limb.

Post-reduction lateral view

A horizontal beam lateral projection is quite easily done without moving the patient out of the wheelchair. The foot rests on a stool or chair. The cassette is placed vertically against the outside of the leg and held in place by the child. If he is not in a wheelchair but on crutches, it is again easier to use a horizontal beam technique on the x-ray table.

Babies

Up to a year old, it is much easier to get a true *PA* than an AP projection of the tibia. Immobilize the baby prone with the compression band across his back. Nurse or mother holds the foot with the ankle extended.

A piece of shaped lead rubber (see Fig. 5, p. 7) will protect her fingers without obscuring the epiphysis of the tibia. Careful positioning is needed to ensure the limb is not rotated. It will be found almost impossible to extend the knee joint fully.

For the *lateral view*, immobilize the leg to be x-rayed with the compression band. Mother holds the baby down and the other leg out of the way (Fig. 59).

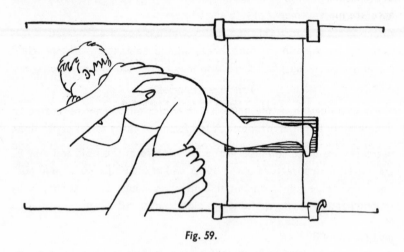

Fig. 59.

Diseases and abnormalities

Acute osteomyelitis. Sarcoma
Osteomyelitis and sarcoma may also occur at the upper end of the tibia. See p. 85. Centre to the presenting swelling.

Bowlegs
Bowlegs is a deformity which can be caused by rickets. Also, a rare disease called achondroplasia may present first as bowlegs in a toddler. An AP view of both legs together on one film is needed. If the child is old enough to sit still and co-operate, use a 30 × 40 cm (15 × 12 in) film to include both knees and ankles, and put a sandbag against the soles of his feet. If he is too young, or unco-operative, lay him down on the table with the compression band across his hips. Mother stands at the end of the table and holds the feet together, toes pointing straight up.

The epiphyses are important for diagnosis, so make sure the ankles and knees will be clearly visible on the film.

Unequal leg lengths

Take one AP film of both legs including both hips and ankles. Exposure factors must take into account the different thicknesses. If surgical correction is contemplated, the child will normally be referred to an orthopaedic centre. The technique of *scanography* is employed for accurate measurements over a period of years.

THE ANKLE AND FOOT

Triple arthrodesis

X-ray examination of the *ankle* is sometimes mistakenly requested to demonstrate triple arthrodesis. It is a fusion of three tarsal bones done at about 12 years of age to relieve foot-drop caused by poliomyelitis and other conditions. It is best demonstrated by a *lateral view of the foot*. Sometimes an oblique view is helpful also.

Fractures

Ankle

Fractures of the lower end of the tibia may have an associated fracture at the upper end of the fibula. The whole length of both bones should be included on a first examination.

Foot

Fractures of the tarsals, metatarsals and phalanges are demonstrated as in adult patients.

Abnormalities of the foot

Hallux valgus

Take one AP view of both feet with the patient standing. Put the cassette on the floor near the end of the x-ray table. The child stands on the cassette and, holding the edge of the table behind him, leans back just enough to allow room for the x-ray tube to be positioned over the feet (Fig. 60). He must not support too much of his weight on his hands.

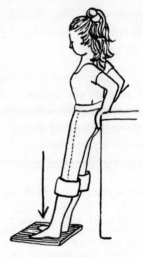

Fig. 60.

Limit the x-ray field to the metatarsals and phalanges. The tarsal bones need not be included. Centre between the big toes, at the level of the metatarsol-phalangeal joints.

Spasmodic flat-foot

Spasmodic flat-foot may be due to an inflammatory lesion of the talo-calcaneal joint, but more often it is due to a congenital bony bridge between the tarsal bones (*tarsal coalition*), occurring in 11–13 year oids.

Talo-calcaneal bar is demonstrated by the axial view for calcaneum with an increase of 5 kv.

Calcaneo-navicular bar is demonstrated by an oblique projection of the mid-foot. From the AP position, the foot is rotated internally until the sole of the foot is at 45° to the cassette. Centre over the head of the 5th metatarsal. Cone to the tarsal bones.

Baby's foot

Fractures

Sit the baby on a pillow or large foam pad on the end of the x-ray table so that his feet are flat on the cassette. Mother puts one arm around him, to hold him in position. With her other hand she holds the leg above the foot to be x-rayed (Fig. 61). A wide piece of Sellotape will keep his toes flat on the film, but not for long! An *oblique view* is taken with a foam wedge under the foot.

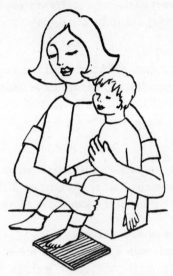

Fig. 61.

Bone age
In babies under 6 months, a film of the foot may be required as well as one of the wrist. Take an AP view of one foot as described above.

Congenital talipes equinus varus (CTEV)
Talipes equino-varus (clubfoot) is a fairly common congenital deformity which may affect one or both feet. The foot is held in plantar flexion; the heel is inverted and the forefoot adducted. Thus, in bilateral cases, the soles face each other.

The diagnosis is apparent at birth and manipulative treatment is started as soon as possible. In between manipulations the foot is held in the corrected position by adhesive strapping, plaster of Paris or a splint. Treatment and supervision usually has to be continued for many months. If conservative treatment fails to overcome the deformity, surgical correction will be necessary. This is advised as early as six weeks of age by some surgeons. A further period of splintage follows the operation.

Opinions vary as to the value of radiography during treatment. Many surgeons dispense with it altogether. Some request films when treatment is finished to assess the degree of correction.

Films taken at intervals during a course of treatment need extremely exact positioning if they are to be comparable for measurements.

AP view (dorsi-plantar)
The usual tube angulation of 25° towards the heel is too great for a baby's foot. The longitudinal arch of the foot necessitating this angulation is not developed until after about 2 years of age. A tilt of 5°–10° is enough, depending on age.

Lateral view
It is sometimes easier to obtain a true lateral projection of a baby's foot by turning the leg inwards (rather than outwards) so that the internal malleolus and inner border of the foot are in contact with the cassette.

Lateral view in maximum dorsi-flexion
A lateral view in maximum dorsi-flexion is sometimes requested. The foot should be held in the corrected position by the orthopaedic house-surgeon (wearing a lead-rubber glove) using a wooden block somewhat larger than the foot to exert pressure on the sole.

A certain number of cases relapse when the child is older. X-ray examination at this time will probably consist of an AP view of both feet and a lateral view of the affected foot. The surgeon may request that these films should be taken with the child standing.

CHAPTER 8

THE SPINE

Children's vertebrae do not suffer from degenerative changes causing the backache for which adults are so often investigated. Therefore it is rarely necessary to take extra views (oblique projections or coned views of lumbo-sacral junction). The routine AP and lateral views are usually sufficient, on initial examination.

INJURIES

Severe injuries

These are fractures and/or dislocations usually caused by road accidents or a fall from a height.

As with an adult patient, x-ray the child on the stretcher if you can do so without moving him. Do not pick him up just because he is small and light. Avoid trying to slide a film and grid under him on the stretcher. If this is not an accident trolley with a film-tray underneath, he must be lifted properly on a canvas and poles by two people to be moved to the x-ray table. When possible, take an AP film first and show it to the radiologist or casualty officer. If it is judged safe to roll the child on his side for the lateral view, do so slowly and carefully 'in one piece'. Stand beside the table facing him, hold the shoulder and hip farthest from you and gently move both towards you at the same rate: thus the alignment of the vertebral column remains undisturbed (Fig. 62).

Alternatively, leave the child supine and use a horizontal beam.

If there is suspected injury to the *cervical spine*, always take one lateral view of that area first and show it to the radiologist or casualty officer before proceeding further.

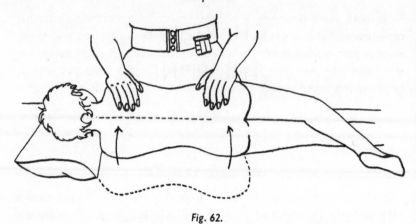

Fig. 62.

Mild injuries

A child may be referred to the x-ray department complaining of pain or stiffness in any part of the spine, maybe with a history of minor injury some days earlier. These patients are usually school-children, and co-operation is no problem. Requests for x-ray examination of toddler's spines are very rare.

THE CERVICAL SPINE

Take AP and lateral views erect. (The use of a grid is optional for the AP projection.) Oblique views and a separate view of C1/C2 area are not necessary on initial examination.

Very young children are better supine as they will not keep still erect.

AP view

The child lies on his back with the chin raised. The head is steadied with a sandbag each side; or mother can hold it straight with two foam pads. Tilt the x-ray tube 5°–10° towards the head.

Lateral view

The child lies on his side. Put a foam pad under his head to bring the cervical spine parallel to the cassette. A 48-in distance compensates for the increased object–film distance.

In both these positions, if the child struggles secure him with the compression band across his hips. In the lateral position you may need another pair of adult hands (father's or nurse's) as well as the compression band (Fig. 63). The head is held firmly on the foam pad with a length of felt orthopaedic bandage by mother (see Fig. 30, p. 45).

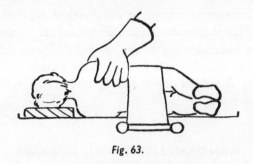

Fig. 63.

THE DORSAL SPINE

AP view
Technique is the same as for an adult.

Lateral view
Ask the child to turn on his side and bend his knees. The arm nearest the table is stretched above his head under the pillow; the uppermost arm is stretched over the top of his head (Fig. 64).

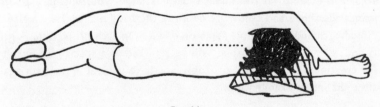

Fig. 64.

A long exposure time, as is sometimes recommended with adults, is not advisable. Very little increase is needed over the AP exposure factors, unless the child is fat or unusually broad across the back. A small child will need *less* exposure for a lateral than for an AP view.

THE LUMBAR SPINE

AP view

It is not necessary to include the sacrum or sacro-iliac joints, unless they are specifically asked for. Use gonad protection for girls as well as boys.

Lateral view

The 5th lumbar vertebra should be easily seen. A separate coned view of the lumbo-sacral junction is not justified except by special request and with the radiologist's approval. A piece of lead rubber can be tucked between a boy's thighs to protect the gonads. For a girl, Sello-tape it on top across the pelvis, making sure it does not obscure the 5th lumbar vertebra.

ABNORMALITIES AND DISEASES

Spina bifida

If your hospital has a maternity unit, you may have to x-ray a newborn baby for spina bifida, a congenital abnormality. It is a condition in which the neural arch of one or more vertebrae and the overlying muscle and skin have failed to close completely during development. The meninges around the cord may protrude through the defect causing a *meningocele*. Part of the cord may protrude also, causing a *myelomeningocele* with nerve damage and paralysis.

It can occur anywhere in the spine but is commonest in the lumbar area. If the lump on the infant's back is large, you will have to use foam pads above and below it; or x-ray the baby prone. Take a lateral film also. Include the whole spine on one film in each projection. A grid is not necessary. These babies will be referred to a specialized hospital for treatment, so you will probably not have to deal with them again after the initial examination.

Spina bifida occulta

A very mild and sometimes symptomless version of the abnormality is spina bifida occulta. The skin has closed normally but the underlying bony arch has not completely fused to form the spinous process. Nerve roots and cord are normal and uninjured but may be adherent and thus pulled as the child grows. This causes interference with the nerve supply to lower limbs and/or sphincters of bladder or rectum. You may be asked to x-ray a 5 or 6 year old who is showing these symptoms. An AP view of the lumbar spine will demonstrate a spina bifida occulta. Bowel preparation is advisable first.

Tuberculosis

Tuberculosis is very rare nowadays in Britain and will not normally be encountered in a general hospital.

However, it is beginning to reappear in areas where there is a large immigrant population from underdeveloped countries. It usually attacks the lower dorsal and lumbar spine, with destruction and collapse of several vertebrae.

Acute osteitis of the spine

Acute osteitis of the spine is a pyogenic infection causing pain and stiffness usually in the lumbar area. Sometimes radiographs are requested to show possible bony erosion.

Scheuermann's disease

Scheuermann's disease is osteochondritis of the dorsal vertebrae. It affects teenagers, mostly girls, and leads to defective growth and a kyphosis. Only a lateral view is required.

Scoliosis

A lateral curvature of the spine (scoliosis) can occur without any known cause, in late childhood and early adolescence. It may deteriorate as the child grows and will need specialist treatment in an orthopaedic centre. For initial diagnosis take an erect view. Use a 35 × 43 cm (14 × 17 in) film with a grid in the chest stand; or stand the child in front of the erect Bucky. A 6-ft focal-film distance is usually employed. Include the spine from C7 to S1. It is important that C7 and the iliac crests are shown on this radiograph. The light beam diaphragm must be opened wide enough to include the epiphyses of the iliac crests because spinal maturity can be assessed from them (Fig. 65).

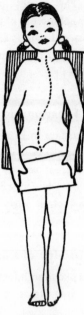

Fig. 65.

At the first examination a lateral projection is also required and maybe an AP projection supine. In the erect position, a girl should hold a piece of lead rubber across the front of the pelvis (*below* the iliac crests) to protect the ovaries.

Torticollis

An acute 'wry-neck' is caused by spasm of the neck muscles. There may or may not be a history of injury. Sometimes an x-ray examination is requested if injury to the cervical spine is suspected. Take the films erect, using the chest stand. Great difficulty will be experienced in positioning for the lateral projection, as the child's head is inclined and rotated to the affected side. Centre to that side, at 6-ft distance, with the child's opposite shoulder touching the cassette.

The resultant radiograph will not look much like a textbook illustration, but the only way to show each vertebra clearly is by several different angled projections. As this condition can occur spontaneously in children without any underlying bony injury, the extra radiation entailed is not justified unless there is grave suspicion of a fracture or dislocation. So if a radiologist's or surgeon's advice is not immediately available, do not keep on repeating lateral views.

Tumours

Tumours of the spine are very rare. Tumours of the cord are rare also but occasionally can be shown radiographically by encroachment on bone. Oblique views are helpful. Myelography is needed for accurate diagnosis.

BABY'S NECK

Request forms asking for x-ray examination of the neck of a baby should not be misinterpreted to mean the cervical spine. The request is most often for a condition called 'stridor' (see p. 37). Radiographic technique is described on pp. 50–51.

CHAPTER 9
THE ABDOMEN

The abdomen extends from the diaphragm to the symphysis pubis: both of these should appear on a radiograph of the abdomen. Probably a larger film than you at first imagine will be found necessary: 24 × 30 cm (12 × 10 in) for a 6-month-old baby, 30 × 40 cm (15 × 12 in) from about 4 years. The younger the child, the larger the body-area taken up by the abdominal cavity.

The usual routine view of the abdomen (which is often somewhat quaintly termed a 'straight' abdomen) is an AP supine projection. A PA projection is employed in certain contrast medium examinations (barium studies of the small bowel, visualization of the ureters in urography) or in infants with gas-filled small gut, to remove these shadows from overlying the kidney outlines. Lateral projections are helpful in localization of abdominal masses and calcifications, and in cases of neonatal intestinal obstruction. Erect films demonstrate air–fluid levels in the gut and free air in the peritoneal space. Decubitis horizontal beam projections serve the same purpose.

Clothing should be removed, but it is not necessary to strip a child naked. Vest and pants can be left on during initial explanations and positioning. For final centring the vest is pulled up to the armpits, and the pants elastic (which is radio-opaque) pulled down to the level of the symphysis pubis. The umbilicus is a fairly accurate centring point at any age.

Gonad protection should always be used on boys but obviously is not possible for girls. Short exposure time is important even for older children: comparatively high kilovoltage (70–80 kV) may be used.

Abdominal radiography of newborn infants is described in Chapter 12.

RADIOGRAPHIC TECHNIQUE

Routine AP view

Babies and toddlers

Set the exposure factors, align the cassette in the Bucky tray with the x-ray beam, close the light beam diaphragm to approximately the required field-size. Ask mother to remove the child's outer clothing and lay him on the table. Help her into a lead coat. Remove the nappy or pants elastic, and tuck the vest out of the way. Adjust the compression band across baby's thighs and knees. Place a rectangle of lead rubber across them also, just below the level of the symphysis pubis: it is less likely to slip from position than a small gonad shield (omit on girls). Mother stands at the head end of the table and holds baby's shoulders firmly flat on the table. She should hold his hands too.

Be as quick as you can, even if baby appears content. He may quite suddenly decide to disapprove of the whole performance.

Exposure time should not exceed 0·04 s to avoid motional blurring. Expose on expiration (watch the rise and fall of his abdomen) as there is least movement of the abdomen at that moment. If he is crying, expose just at the end of a yell.

Older children

From about 3 or 4 years onwards the compression band is not necessary over the legs, if the child will lie still and is not upset. Mother can stand at the head end of the table as before and hold his hands up beside his shoulders. Ask him to 'keep his tummy still' if he is too young to hold his breath, and use 0·04 s exposure time.

The upper border of the abdomen is an inch or two below the level of the nipples at this age. It varies with the age and build of the child. Experience will soon teach you where to set the upper limit of the x-ray field. A boy's gonads should not appear on an abdomen film.

Lateral view

Babies and toddlers

A child with intestinal obstruction or an abdominal mass (the usual reasons for lateral views of the abdomen at this age) will probably be quite ill, and not inclined to offer much resistance. Turn him on his side; mother can hold him steady with one hand on his shoulder and the other on his hip. It is important he should lie in a true lateral position; explain to mother that she must not allow him to roll forwards.

Older children

A child old enough to co-operate should be positioned as for a lateral view of the spine, except that the legs are straight. This position is not easily maintained: so to prevent him rolling forwards into an oblique position, mother or nurse holds the legs about knee level to steady him. Gonad protection for boys is provided by a piece of flexible lead rubber laid across the upper thigh.

Erect AP view

Older children

Over the age of about 5 years, a child can stand in front of an upright Bucky, or grid cassette in the chest stand, for an erect view of the abdomen. To steady himself tell him to hold the bottom edge of the Bucky behind him. If he is too ill to stand, he should be transported on a stretcher, not a chair, to the x-ray department. It is then a simple matter to sit him upright on the stretcher with his legs over the side. A foam pad under his bottom will raise him enough to ensure that the whole abdomen is included on the radiograph. His knees should be wide apart. Prop a small piece of lead rubber upright for gonad protection of a boy (Fig. 66).

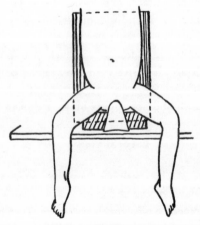

Fig. 66.

Babies

Whatever method is in use for erect chest radiography can be employed for erect abdomen films also. It is only necessary to raise the baby higher by sitting him astride a 45° foam block on the seat. The Velcro strap goes across his lower thighs. Gonad protection is better left off, unless it can be secured in place with great accuracy. Nurse or mother, standing behind or beside baby, holds the arms upright, not by the elbows but at shoulder level, thus holding the trunk straight also. The adult's hands must be well above the upper limit of the x-ray field (Fig. 67). A very small baby cannot safely be held upright in this way by a nurse wearing lead–rubber gloves, though it may be possible to wear them for holding an older, larger baby.

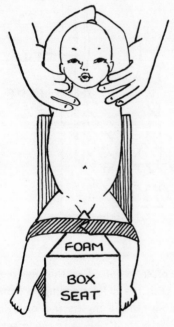

Fig. 67.

If chest radiographs are normally taken supine, some method of seating baby upright, with his legs out of the way, will have to be improvised. It is no good trying to take an erect view of the abdomen with baby's legs on the same level as his bottom: the thighs will be superimposed over the lower abdomen.

The simplest method is that described on p. 143 (See also Fig. 75, p. 139) utilizing the detachable step on the screening table. If the baby is over 6 months it will be necessary to raise both child and cassette slightly higher, in order to leave room for the extra length of leg. A rectangular foam pad under both the cassette and the 45° foam pad will achieve this (Fig. 68). A grid is used.

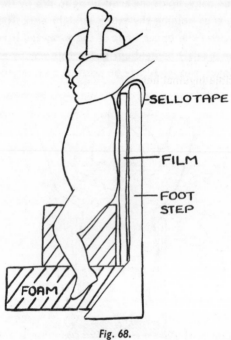

Fig. 68.

2–5 years

Erect films are not often required in this age-group. They are most conveniently taken with the child standing in front of a grid-cassette (30 × 40 cm, 12 × 10 in) in the chest stand, on a firm flat-seated chair. A Velcro strap around the child's hips and the lower part of the cassette will help to keep him in an AP position. The arms are held up at shoulder level, as described above for babies.

Decubitis films with horizontal beam

These projections will normally be employed only on babies or children who are too ill for erect films. Restraint will be unnecessary in this case, and the technique is the same as for adult patients. A lateral decubitus projection is easier than an AP projection on young children.

PATHOLOGY

Intestinal obstruction

In the newborn infant, intestinal obstruction is nearly always due to a congenital abnormality (see Chapter 12, p. 134). In slightly older babies, up to about 2 years, the commonest causes are as follows:

(i) an irreducible inguinal hernia;

(ii) adhesions following an attack of peritonitis or an operation;

(iii) *intussusception*: a condition in which a segment of intestine telescopes into the following segment in the same way as a tuck is made in a sleeve to shorten it (Fig. 69). Peristalsis increases in an effort to overcome this, but only succeeds in making it worse.

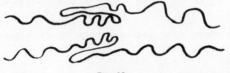

Fig. 69.

The diagnosis of intussusception is often made clinically and treated surgically without the assistance of radiology. (But see also p. 126.)

In older children, the usual cause of obstruction is adhesions.

If strangulation follows obstruction, surgery is urgently needed to save the child's life.

Erect or decubitus horizontal-beam projections are normally required as well as a supine AP view, in any case of suspected intestinal obstruction.

Abdominal pain

Children with vague abdominal pain of unspecified cause are often sent for x-ray examination. One supine film usually is sufficient. An erect view may be requested. A chest film may be required also, as the abdominal pain may be caused by a lower lobe pneumonia.

Appendicitis

The diagnosis of appendicitis is a clinical one, but radiography may be requested to exclude other abnormalities. Occasionally a faecolith is demonstrated in the appendix.

Post-operatively, the possible complications include sub-phrenic abscess (see Chapter 2, p. 39) and pelvic abscess, either of which may necessitate x-ray examination.

Trauma

A road accident is the usual cause. Any abdominal organ may be injured and bleed; the intestine may be ruptured causing pneumoperitoneum. Erect or decubitus horizontal-beam projections should be taken as well as the supine view.

Abdominal masses

Abdominal masses are rare, but need urgent investigation when they occur. As the mass may be a hydronephrosis, hydroureter, or a malignant tumour involving or displacing the renal tract, excretion urography is always requested. Therefore the initial examination consists of only one supine AP view of the abdomen possibly also a lateral view.

Calcification

Any evidence of calcification in an abdominal radiograph, the exact site of which is in doubt, can be more exactly localized by a lateral film than by the inspiration–expiration films usual in an adult. Stones in the renal tract are fairly uncommon; gallstones are extremely rare in children.

Swallowed foreign bodies

Babies and young children have a tendency to swallow a wide variety of small objects. The commonest are coins, marbles, hairgrips, pins and bits of toys. Mostly they go straight through the alimentary tract and cause no harm, but occasionally they get stuck on the way.

The usual sites of obstruction in the oesophagus are: just above the level of the sternal notch; midway, at the level of the left main bronchus; at the lower end just above the stomach. Most foreign bodies reaching the stomach will continue on their course without difficulty. However, long thin objects such as a hairgrip, may stick in the duodenal loop or terminal ileum.

The first radiograph taken to confirm the presence of a swallowed foreign body and to localize its position should include the entire alimentary tract from pharynx to anus on one film. A 35 × 43 cm (17 × 14 in) cassette is used. The child's head is turned to one side, for better visualization of the pharynx and upper oesophagus. If the child is too big to fit on one film, the 35 × 43 cm film should include from the anus upwards and a separate 18 × 24 cm (10 × 8 in) film is taken immediately after, from the base of the skull down, with the child supine and the head in the lateral position.

Some plastic objects are surprisingly opaque. If the mother has had the forethought to bring along another similar object (e.g. button, 'Lego' brick, etc.) it is a good idea to x-ray it to assess its radio-opacity.

Objects lodged in the oesophagus are retrieved by endoscopy under general anaesthetic. A second radiograph should always be taken immediately before the child is anaesthetized, to confirm that the object has not progressed to the stomach or been vomited.

Children who have swallowed pins, hairgrips or similar potentially dangerous objects are admitted to hospital for observation in view of the possibility of perforation. Those in whom swallowed coins, marbles, etc., are first located in the stomach are not usually hospitalized, but are x-rayed again a week or so later to confirm that the object has been passed.

If the swallowed object appears to be still in the stomach after a week, a lateral film of the upper abdomen will localize it to either the stomach or the small gut.

CHAPTER 10
THE URINARY TRACT

EXCRETION UROGRAPHY

Investigations of the urinary tract constitute a large proportion of the radiological examinations of children. Indications for performing excretion urography include:

(i) urinary tract infections;
(ii) enuresis;
(iii) haematuria;
(iv) certain categories of abdominal pain;
(v) abdominal mass;
(vi) trauma to the region of the loin.

An intravenous urogram (IVU) is routinely performed on infants with congenital malformations of the external genitalia, imperforate anus, and myelomeningocele. There is an associated malformation of the urinary tract in a percentage of these patients.

There is a great deal of varied opinion among radiologists as to the number, timing, and area of radiographs constituting an ideal excretion urogram. Continuous supervision by the radiologist, from the control film onwards, is to be preferred over any set routine. Consequently this chapter is confined to those specific points wherein the renal tract radiography of children differs from that of adults.

Routine procedure
Preparation
It is usual to give some form of *laxative* such as Senokot, the type and dosage being decided by the radiologist. Routine *sedation* of small children does not appear to be usual in children's hospitals, but some

x-ray departments may consider it advantageous. It has the disadvantage of adding several hours to the time spent by mother and child in the hospital and the necessity of providing somewhere quiet for the child to lie down when it begins to take effect. For babies under 6 months, sedation and a preparatory enema may be considered helpful.

With the relatively high doses of contrast media in use now, *dehydration* has become much less important. In children under 5 years, restricting fluids can be positively unhelpful in that the discomfort of thirst results in constant crying, so large amounts of air are swallowed. Older children can be instructed not to drink anything for 2–3 hours before the appointment, or whatever length of time the radiologist considers necessary, but this may well be omitted with the smaller ones.

Control film

One film is adequate for all but tall teenagers: 18 × 24 cm (10 × 8 in) for infants, 24 × 30 cm (12 × 10 in) for babies (6 months onwards), 30 × 40 cm (15 × 12 in) over about 4 years. The choice of exposure factors will depend on whether the child can hold his breath. Slight inspiration is the easiest to hold: rehearse it a few times. The competent breath-holder will probably be over 6–7 years. The exposure factors can be adapted from those used for a small thin adult, kilovoltage in the 60–68 range to obtain good soft tissue detail and contrast. Under that age, low kilovoltage may have to be sacrificed in order to reduce the time: 70–85 kV may be used. The maximum time for babies, in whom crying will increase the likelihood of movement, is 0·04 s. As ordinary shallow breathing does not cause anything like as much movement of the kidneys as of the intestines, this can be increased to 0·06 or 0·07 s for 4–5 year olds. The short time essential for a plain film of the abdominal gastro-intestinal tract is not quite so critical for the renal tract.

The radiologist should be shown the control film in order to assess whether the preparation has been adequate, or whether further preparation in the form of a Veripaque or other enema is necessary, or perhaps another course of Senokot or similar laxative and another appointment.

Contrast medium

Conray 280, Hypaque 45, Urografin 290 or 325 (Urovision) are commonly used. The dose is determined by mililitre per kilogramme body-weight. High dose urography entails 2 ml per kg. As a rough guide 15 ml may be used up to 6 months, 30 ml thereafter; 40 ml for fat children or those with a high blood urea.

The usual anti-reaction drugs, oxygen supply and a paediatric resuscitation kit must always be at hand.

The injection

Contrast medium should always be injected intravenously, not intra-muscularly. The manufacture of 'butterfly' needles has greatly facilitated this. A vein can usually be found, if not in the arm, in the foot or back of the hand, or in the case of a small baby, in the scalp. The child must be warned immediately beforehand. A firm grip on the arm or leg is preferable to the use of a tourniquet; release your grip but keep your hand in place once the vein is punctured, as the child may try to jerk the limb away from the doctor. If the injection site is the anterior elbow, most children will instinctively try to flex the joint at the moment of injection, so make sure the arm is immovably fixed in extension: hold the child's hand as well as his upper arm. It is helpful if a second radio-grapher, or a nurse, can stand by for the injection, ready to hold the child's legs if he suddenly gets upset and starts to struggle.

If it is to be a scalp-vein injection, it is better that a nurse who is used to the technique should hold the baby's head rather than a radio-grapher. Persuade the mother, kindly, that she would be better off outside the room while this is done.

It is wise, in any case, to ask the house surgeon whether he minds the mother being present for the injection. (If he is new to the job it may put him off, and venepuncture of a child is never easy.) Ask the mother also whether she prefers to stay or leave the room. If she does not want to stay, a nurse or other member of staff should stand the other side of the table from the doctor, and distract the child's attention by talking about his family or school or anything else that will engage his interest.

After the injection a relative or nurse must stay with the child for the entire examination, in case of a delayed reaction. Small children should be read to, so that they do not get restless.

Post-injection films

It is difficult to demonstrate kidney outlines in younger children and babies, because of the relatively small amount of peri-renal fat and the frequent presence of intestinal gas shadows. The fizzy drink technique is often successfully employed to distend the stomach sufficiently for the kidneys to be clearly seen through it. However, it is not always possible to persuade children to drink enough (some do not like fizz) or, if they do, the gas will almost certainly obscure the lower renal tract in subsequent films. With the high dose of contrast medium usually given nowadays, a localized film of the kidney area taken immediately or at 1 or 2 min after the injection should show a nephrogram of both kidneys even through bowel shadows. Because of the difficulty in visualizing the kidney outlines on the control film this nephrogram may be the only way of demonstrating them. It is important that it should be attempted, as the assessment of kidney size, and growth in follow-up examinations, is essential in the diagnosis and management of children with urinary tract disorders.

The timing of subsequent films is at the radiologist's discretion. A further film of the kidney area may be taken at 8, 10, 12 or 15 min. At least one full-length film is included at perhaps 20 or 25 min (15 min for a baby). Most radiologists like an after-micturition film, but otherwise no separate radiograph of the bladder is necessary.

Compression is not usually employed; instead some radiologists like the table to be tilted head down after the first film until the full-length film is due. The number of radiographs is kept to a minimum, especially for follow-up examinations done to assess the effect of medical or surgical treatment. Because of this, radiography should be of the highest possible quality.

A *prone film* on older children is useful to demonstrate the ureters, if taken immediately after the child turns over. The prone position may also demonstrate a hydronephrotic kidney, of which the calyces are hardly visible in a supine film. The contrast medium will pool in the more anterior renal pelvis.

An *erect film* may show a hydronephrotic kidney even more successfully.

A *lateral film* taken between 15 and 30 min is very useful in localizing an abdominal tumour and in some departments is routinely taken in

every case of an abdominal mass. Excretion urography is the first
investigation in all such patients.

Modifications

Babies

With babies, who normally have a fairly large amount of small bowel
gas, it can be helpful to have them nursed prone for some hours prior
to examination. If they are then bottle-fed immediately after the
injection it has a soothing effect and the amount of swallowed air helps
to distend the stomach. A compression band, not too tightly applied,
over the back, helps to push the intestinal gas to the sides of the abdomen
and keep the baby in position. The first film can be taken prone: if
visualization of the kidneys is not good, turn the baby supine once an
ounce or so of the feed has been taken. This acts as a plug to keep the
air in the stomach when baby lies on his back. The stomach will distend
further with swallowed air and the kidneys may be better visualized on
a subsequent supine film. The Potter-Bucky is used even for infants.

Follow-up examinations

Follow-up urograms are done to assess the effect of treatment, and
regularly at yearly or half-yearly intervals on children under periodic
review. Two films (plus a control film of course) are usually taken:
an early nephrogram to demonstrate kidney growth, and a full-length
film of the whole renal tract at 20 or 25 min.

Zonograms

Though often routinely done in adults, zonograms are to be avoided
when possible in children, as the radiation dose may well be higher.
Careful bowel preparation and the obtaining of a good nephrogram as
described above, should reduce to an absolute minimum the necessity
for zonography simply to show kidney outline.

'Non-functioning' kidney

The visualization of only one kidney on a urogram means either congenital absence of the other, or that pathology has destroyed its functioning or is causing it to function very slowly. A hydronephrotic
kidney may not appear radiographically for several hours. If such is

suspected; further films should be taken at 1, 2 and 6 h, possibly prone and/or erect.

Trauma

When injury occurs in the region of the loin, most often from a road accident, emergency excretion urography may be necessary to assess the indications for surgery and the condition of the uninjured kidney.

Parents

When the appointment is made for excretion urography, the procedure, the importance of adhering to the preparation instructions and the necessity for an injection (and sedation) must all be carefully explained —preferably out of hearing of the child if he is very young or nervous. Explain also that the examination may take quite a time. After the first film is taken, parents often ask how many more will be necessary. It is wisest not to give a definite answer, but to say it depends on what the doctor sees on each film as it is taken. Abnormalities may be discovered which necessitate more films than usual. You will avoid alarming the parents if they do not realize this.

Pathology

Congenital abnormalities

There are many varieties, some of which are:

(i) *ectopic kidney*: because of a developmental error one kidney is situated lower in the abdomen;

(ii) *horseshoe kidney*: where the lower poles of both kidneys are joined by a band of renal tissue;

(iii) *unilateral agenesis*: one kidney is absent (bilateral is incompatible with survival);

(iv) *duplication*: many varieties, including duplex kidney and/or duplex ureter, unilateral or bilateral;

(v) *congenital hydronephrosis and hydroureter*: presenting as an abdominal mass in an infant.

Infection

Infections of the urinary tract are common in childhood. If left untreated, recurrent episodes often result in damage to the kidneys (renal scarring) and eventual renal failure. Infection is frequently associated with anatomical abnormalities of the urinary tract and with the physiological abnormality of reflux of urine up one or both ureters.

Hydronephrosis and hydroureter
This condition is caused by obstruction of the flow of urine at any point in the tract and is the commonest disorder of the urinary tract in childhood. The causes and sites of obstruction are many. If unilateral, the obstruction is sited above the bladder; if bilateral, it is in or below it. The tract above the obstruction becomes dilated and its function impaired. The common sites of obstruction are:

the pelvi-uretic junction; the junction of ureter and bladder;
at the bladder neck or in the urethra, where abnormal mucosal folds (*urethral valve*) can occur in boys.

Depending on how long the condition has been present before diagnosis, there will be a greater or lesser degree of dilatation of the ureter and the renal pelvis. The treatment is surgical relief of the obstruction.

Calculi
A calculus may occur anywhere in the urinary tract, but most often in the pelvis and calyces of one kidney, when it is called a 'staghorn' calculus.

Diverticula of bladder
Often diverticula are not seen on excretion urography and not diagnosed until a micturating cystogram is done.

Malignancy
Nephroblastoma or Wilms' tumour is a highly malignant tumour of embryonic origin, originating in the kidney tissue and presenting usually between 1 and 3 years.

Neuroblastoma is also a malignant tumour of embryonic origin. It does not arise in the urinary tract, but an abdominal neuroblastoma is in close proximity to the kidney. It arises in the adrenal gland, or in the sympathetic nerve chain in the posterior abdominal wall. (It can also arise from the latter site in the thorax.)

Chest radiographs will be needed to exclude secondary deposits, possibly a skeletal survey also.

MICTURATING CYSTOGRAPHY

This examination is performed in children mainly to investigate the presence of reflux of urine from the bladder up the ureter(s). This may occur either during the retrograde filling of the bladder, or during micturition. Reflux is fairly common in children, and is the cause of much trouble in the urinary tract. Abnormalities of the bladder itself (diverticula, etc.) and of the urethra (congenital valves, etc.) are also demonstrated.

Sedation
Sedation is usually employed for children under about 6 years of age. It may be found convenient to admit them as day cases, in order that sedation and catheterization can be carried out in the ward. X-ray examination should follow as soon as possible after catheterization.

The examination
The screening table is left in the horizontal position, with footstep and handles for the patient in place. Some radiologists conduct the whole examination with the patient supine, but, when examining older children, many prefer to bring the table upright, once the bladder has been filled. Babies and very young children are always examined in the supine position. Cellulose wadding is used instead of a urine receptacle. Legs are immobilized in tubular elastic bandage.

A parent or nurse should be with the child throughout for comfort and encouragement, as it is not a pleasant experience. When the child is lying on the table, the spigot should be removed from the catheter and the bladder drained into a kidney dish. It is advisable to remove his shoes and socks now also, in case of splashes later. The catheter is then connected to a paediatric drip-set, the other end of which is connected to a 250-ml bottle of Urografin 150, or similar contrast medium for infusion. Care must be taken that this is done as aseptically as possible as there is always a risk of introducing infection into a catheterized bladder. The radiologist then screens briefly at intervals as the bladder fills. If reflux is noted, he will take films with the undercouch tube. When the bladder is judged to be full, the drip infusion is stopped and the catheter removed.

The rest of the examination must be executed speedily, as once the catheter is removed, the child may not be able to control micturition. A plastic or disposal urine bottle is used for boys, held by the patient if he is old enough. If not, a potty can be held by a nurse wearing a lead–rubber glove. A little boy will 'wee' into a potty more readily than into a bottle. Cellulose wadding, a kidney dish or a plastic funnel, connected by tube to a bucket, can be used for girls. The funnel provided with a rectal wash-out pack is suitable. The edges are a bit sharp and need some padding (gauze swabs or similar) Sellotaped over them. If possible, the receptacle is positioned before the table is tilted upright, in case the child starts micturition immediately.

Everything should be set in readiness for swift changing of the cassettes, and of the exposure factors if necessary (for lateral or oblique projections) during the micturition series of radiographs. Some radiologists use a serial film as for duodenal cap series, some use two or three split 24 × 30 cm (12 × 10 in) films.

If a micturating cystogram and an excretion urogram are to be performed on a child on the same day, the cystogram should be done first. If the urogram is done first, the contrast medium may not have been completely excreted by the kidneys before the cystogram is performed.

Sometimes a non-functioning kidney, or part of a duplex system not visualized on the urogram, will be demonstrated with startling clarity by a reflux flood of contrast filling ureter, renal pelvis and calyces.

Babies

An infant's naso-gastric tube can be utilized as a catheter for babies. The bladder is filled from a 50-ml syringe instead of the drip infusion method. If the bladder is completely filled, the removal of the catheter should start off micturition. If not, a drink, or pressure on the lower abdomen or a warm compress can be tried.

Expression cystography

In some hospitals it is usual to perform an expression cystogram rather than micturating cystography on small children under 2 or 3 years. Under general anaesthetic the child is catheterized and the bladder filled by syringe, under fluoroscopic control if possible. When the bladder is judged to be full, a cassette is placed under the pelvis and the catheter removed. The surgeon presses on the bladder to initiate micturition.

RETROGRADE PYELOGRAPHY

Retrograde pyelography is not often considered necessary. Abnormal anatomy is demonstrated with a sharper radiographic outline than in excretion urography, as the contrast medium is not diluted by urine. The level of an obstruction in a ureter will be demonstrated, and the state of a ureter draining a hydronephrotic kidney.

Catheterization for retrograde pyelography follows cystoscopy, as in adults, but the x-ray examination also is done under general anaesthetic. Therefore, it is usually performed by the surgeon in the operating theatre. Although ideally retrograde filling of the kidney pelvis should be conducted under fluoroscopic control, this is possible only if a mobile fluoroscopic unit is available in theatre.

The contrast medium used is the same as for adults: only 2 ml is injected initially. One full-length radiograph is then taken. This may be sufficient, or it may be decided to inject a further millilitre or two and take a second film.

It is often useful to take a delayed film, at 20 min or so, for assessment of drainage.

NEPHROSTOGRAM

An obstruction at the pelvi-ureteric junction results eventually in a dilated renal pelvis. After relief of the obstruction, the operation of pyeloplasty is sometimes performed. Part of the dilated pelvis is removed and the ureter is anastomosed at a different site. While the anastomosis is healing, the renal pelvis is drained by a short catheter (nephrostomy tube) through the loin.

Before the nephrostomy can be closed and urine allowed to drain normally again, the surgeon must be sure that there is no leak at the anastomosis and that the ureter is patent.

Under fluoroscopic control, the radiologist injects 5–10 ml of Hypaque 25, Retroconray or similar contrast medium through the nephrostomy tube to fill the renal pelvis. Films are taken as required with the undercouch tube.

The nephrostomy tube is then closed off with a clip and the patient returns to the ward or waiting room. He remains sitting upright for 30 min. An AP view of the renal tract is then taken to assess drainage down the ureter. This film is shown to the radiologist who may decide that another should be taken after a further interval. The clip is removed when the examination is finished.

CHAPTER 11

THE GASTRO-INTESTINAL TRACT

BARIUM SWALLOWS AND MEALS

Fluoroscopic studies of the oesophagus in children are almost entirely confined to the infant age group. After the first year, almost the only reason for a barium swallow examination is the assessment of damage to a small child's oesophagus after accidental swallowing of caustic poison. This is done some weeks later, after the burns on the mouth have healed.

Persistent abnormal vomiting, failure to thrive, stridor (see p. 37) with no known respiratory cause, and choking over feeds are the usual reasons for requesting fluoroscopic investigation of babies.

Pathology

Hiatus hernia
The same abnormality as that found in adults, hiatus hernia is quite common in babies and causes vomiting after feeds.

Abnormalities of the swallowing mechanism
These may have a neurological origin.

Vascular ring
Abnormal anatomy of the bloodvessels around the oesophagus and trachea (a vascular ring) may compress the trachea and cause stridor.

Pyloric stenosis
A congenital narrowing of the pylorus is a fairly common defect. It is frequently diagnosed clinically, without radiology.

'H-type' tracheo-oesophageal fistula

A rare variant of tracheo-oesophageal fistula (see p. 133) is that in which an otherwise normal trachea and oesophagus are joined by a fistula (thus making an H). There is no accompanying atresia of the oesophagus (see p. 133). The infant, a week or two old, will choke over attempts to feed.

Failure to thrive

The causes of failure to thrive are many and various. Vomiting after feeding is one cause in infancy; malabsorption syndrome, a malfunction of the small bowel, may be the cause in a young child.

Investigations

Suspected *vascular ring, swallowing disorders,* or *tracheo-oesophageal fistula,* are investigated by opaque *swallows.* The last two conditions require videotape recording in addition to fluoroscopy.

Hiatus hernia needs a barium *meal* examination, though the request is usually for barium swallow. The stomach has to be filled to demonstrate the hernia.

Failure to thrive may be investigated by barium *swallow* (in infants), barium *meal* or *follow-through* examination.

Parents

The question of whether or not a parent accompanies a child undergoing fluoroscopy is a decision for the radiologist. Generally it is best to allow a mother to look after and feed a baby over 3–4 months and to be with a small child under 5 years for reassurance. A nurse may be better to manage an infant under 3 months, rather than a mother if it is her first baby.

Barium amounts

The amount of barium sulphate suspension necessary at different ages is decided by the radiologist; some require more than others. Micropaque (or similar) is diluted 50% with sterile water for babies under 6 months, after that age they can take it neat. Gastrografin should be used with care in babies and young children as it may cause dehydration.

The extra barium given for a follow-through examination may be diluted 50% with water. Suggestions for amounts:

Baby   1–2 oz bottle, diluted 50%, for swallow, meal and follow-through

1 year   2 or 3 spoonfuls neat Micropaque first, then 1 oz (30 ml) diluted

2 years 1 or 2 oz neat Micropaque first, then 2 oz (50–60 ml) diluted

4 years 1 or 2 oz neat Micropaque first, then 3 oz (100 ml) diluted

8 years 1 or 2 oz neat Micropaque first, then 6 oz (200 ml) diluted

Technique

Bottle-fed babies

The bottle is warmed by standing it in a jug of hot water shortly before needed; it should be shaken every now and then. You can judge when it is warm enough by shaking out a few drops on the back of your hand. The hole in the teat will need to be enlarged with a scalpel blade.

The time for the examination should coincide with the time a feed is due so that baby will be hungry. The taste of barium does not seem to matter to infants and they usually take it without trouble.

A nurse or the mother should see to the feeding during the examination. Show her how to hold the baby and the bottle in the way most helpful to the radiologist. Standing at the top end of the table, she should hold the bottle in her right hand, and the baby's arms above his head with her left hand. The wearing of lead–rubber gloves makes this almost impossible. Instead, two pieces of lead rubber are carefully placed on the table leaving a space between for baby's head (Fig. 70). These protect nurse's hands from radiation from the undercouch tube. They must never slip out of place under the baby and obscure the radiologist's view. When it is necessary to stop feeding, nurse tilts the bottle lower than level so that no barium reaches the teat, but the teat is left in baby's mouth. He can continue sucking, which prevents the crying that would result from withdrawal of the teat.

The radiologist holds the legs and controls the rotation of the baby as he wishes. In some hospitals a form of 'brat-board' is used for immobilization. Most radiologists screen a baby prone during the examination and some consider a brat-board to be a nuisance in this manoeuvre.

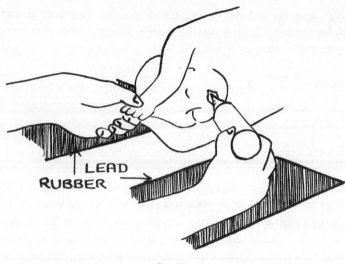

LEAD
RUBBER

Fig. 70.

Others find it a help. A length of tubular elasticated bandage around the legs can be helpful. The grid is not used for babies under 6 months.

Care should be taken to ensure than an infant does not get chilled. Vest and nappy should be left on, but a shawl or blanket will need to be removed. An 'Inco-pad' folded over a thin piece of foam of appropriate size makes a convenient mattress. A newborn or very young infant, or one who is nursed in an incubator, must have a layer of gamgee or cottonwool both under and over him during the entire examination.

Tracheo-oesophageal fistula
If the examination is for tracheo-oesophageal fistula, or if there is any other reason for expecting that some of the swallowed medium might reach the lungs, Dionosil (either oily or acqueous) is used instead of barium. Gastrografin is definitely not used; it has a damaging effect on lung tissue.

Dionosil is sold in bottles of 20 ml. A teat with greatly enlarged hole can be put straight on the bottle: there is no need to transfer the Dionosil to a feeding-bottle. A sucker, plugged in and ready for use with correct size catheter attached, and an oxygen cylinder with infant size fittings, must be to hand in the screening room. Test both before you send for the baby. If he is coming in an incubator, check that a correct plug-socket or adaptor is available and warm the room.

Toddlers

Over 6 months of age children should be starved for 4 h before the examination.

A one year old can be spoon-fed; a two year old may prefer a cup. When the appointment is made, ask mother how he is fed at home. If he drinks from a spouted beaker, she might like to bring his own along with him. He will be happier drinking from his own cup than from a strange one. It must be possible to drink from it lying down.

It is helpful to have a nurse to assist as well as mother at this age. Mother can spoon-feed him, not an easy job if he is lying prone. Nurse can see that he lies in the correct position for the radiologist.

If mother proves inadequate to the task of getting the barium swallowed, she and nurse should change places. If you then hold the child's head firmly so that he cannot turn it to one side, while mother holds the rest of him, nurse can use the time-honoured method of getting medicine down a child. The barium is tipped from a spoon into his mouth as he opens it to yell in protest. His mouth is then held closed until he swallows.

This manoeuvre should be accompanied by a non-stop, encouraging, soothing line of chat to reassure both child and mother that it is not as drastic a procedure as it appears.

3–5 years

After about 3 years of age, flexible straws are useful, as small children usually enjoy drinking through a straw. There are various flavoured brands of barium sulphate suspension on the market. Orange squash can be added to Micropaque if preferred. Some radiologists like an effervescent preparation of barium (such as Baritop).

A child of this age may have to be persuaded to drink, but generally speaking there is rarely any difficulty. The spoilt child of doting parents is the only one likely to refuse. It is advisable to arrange for a nurse to take charge of such a child for the examination, and to ask mother to wait outside.

Small bowel follow-through

The onset of coeliac disease is from 1 to 2 years. Any child from that age on who is failing to thrive may be suspected of suffering from this or some other form of malabsorption, and be referred for small bowel barium examination.

The child should starve for 6 h (a baby for 4 h); Micropaque (or similar) is used, diluted 50% with water. Some radiologists add 1–2 ml of Gastrografin to the Micropaque. It should be kept overnight in a refrigerator: it travels faster when cold. Also you can pretend it is a special kind of ice-cream.

After the correct amount of barium has been swallowed, the child lies on his right side for 10–15 min. A film of the whole abdomen is taken prone at 20 min. Thereafter the radiologist decides at what intervals the subsequent films should be taken, possibly every 20 min or half-hour until the caecum is reached. The last film is taken with a foam pad doubled up under the right iliac fossa, to separate the loops of small gut and allow the terminal ilieum to be seen.

The technique of jejunal biopsy (see below) is also employed for diagnosis of malabsorption.

Older children

Children over 5 years are dealt with as adults. They may not like the barium but they normally drink it with no trouble.

The usual reason for examination of this age-group is a suspected peptic ulcer or duodenal ulcer. These are not nearly as common in children as in adults.

An odd and very rare finding is a hairball (trichobezoar). Small girls who habitually chew the ends of their long hair can end up with quite severe symptoms of wasting. A hairball can enlarge to occupy the whole of the stomach interior before its presence is suspected.

JEJUNAL BIOPSY

One way of diagnosing malabsorption syndrome is to obtain a biopsy of jejunal mucosa. It is possible to do this by passing a tube either through the mouth or nose via the stomach and into the jejunum. At the swallowed end of the tube is a small capsule by means of which a biopsy can be taken.

The child is x-rayed simply to determine when the capsule is in the jejunum. This may be done by fluoroscopy or by a radiograph of the upper abdomen. A time should be agreed with the ward so that the child is not kept waiting around (if he is very young he will probably be sedated).

If a radiograph is taken it need include only the upper abdomen (stomach, duodenum and jejunum) so as to avoid irradiating the gonads.

BARIUM ENEMA

Barium enema examination is not often requested in children. The reasons for the investigation tend to occur in three main age-groups as follows:

(i)   intestinal obstruction in the newborn;
(ii) intussusception in the toddler;
(iii) chronic constipation, rectal bleeding, or recurrent attacks of diarrhoea in the older child.

Pathology
Hirschsprung's disease
The commonest cause of large bowel obstruction in the newborn is Hirschsprung's disease, which may be provisionally diagnosed from the initial radiographs of the abdomen. The diagnosis is confirmed and the extent of the abnormality assessed by barium enema. The examination is performed as an emergency measure before surgery to relieve the obstruction. (See also p. 135.)

Occasionally an older child who is chronically constipated may be referred for barium enema to exclude a mild form of the disease. The causes of chronic constipation are usually wrong diet and faulty toilet training.

Colonic polyp
Rectal bleeding is most often caused by a colonic polyp. A double-contrast enema is performed for diagnosis. A small amount of barium is used to coat the intestinal walls, followed by air insufflation.

Chronic ulcerative colitis

A rare disease in childhood, chronic ulcerative colitis has no known cause. The child suffers from severe diarrhoea. The bowel outline appears quite smooth without the normal haustrations. An after-evacuation film is important to show the mucosal pattern.

Intussusception

Occasionally a barium enema may be considered helpful in localizing the site of an intussusception (see Chapter 9, p. 105). Some radiologists undertake a barium enema which will not only demonstrate the condition but may also reduce it, thus avoiding the need for surgery. There are widely differing points of view on this subject.

Preparation

When *Hirschsprung's disease* or *intussusception* is suspected no preparation whatever is done.

Double-contrast enema for diagnosis and location of *a polyp* needs extremely thorough preparation. Ideally the examination should be performed on a completely empty colon. Most radiologists have their own preferred methods of preparation. These may include a combination of orally administered medicine and a series of enemas (Veripaque, phosphate or other). The routine may take 2 or 3 days so the child is often admitted to hospital for this period.

Preparation for a child thought to be suffering from *ulcerative colitis* will be decided on possibly after discussion between the radiologist and clinician. It must be very carefully carried out because of the already inflamed state of the bowel.

Equipment

It is a good idea to keep a box packed with the necessary items for an infant's barium enema. A selection of disposable catheters of various sizes for children might also be included.

A suggested list of contents follows.

Infants   Two 50-ml syringes with nozzles (irrigating type)
Rubber disposable catheters sizes 8, 10, 12
Two 100-ml bottles of normal saline
Narrow adhesive tape
Tubular elasticated bandage, 10 cm (4 in) wide, (for legs)

Children   Disposable rubber or soft plastic catheters, sizes 12–20
Two 500-ml packs of normal saline

In addition a potty or small bedpan is useful.

The usual equipment for adult enemas is also needed as follows:

(i)   enema can, tubing and stand;
(ii)   disposable connectors (to join tubing and catheter);
(iii)   swabs and lubricating jelly;
(iv)   2 Spencer Wells forceps or clips;
(v)   'Inco' pads or cellulose wadding;
(vi)   Higginson's syringe for air insufflation;
(vii)   plastic bucket, if large amounts of barium are generally used.

Technique

Barium enemas for babies are mixed with equal parts of Micropaque (or similar) and normal saline, not ordinary water. In some x-ray departments this applies to all children's barium enemas. From 100 to 300 ml ($\frac{1}{2}$ pint) is made up for infants and older babies; 1 litre or 1–1$\frac{1}{2}$ pints for a child. It should be warmed before use. There must be no air bubbles in the barium mixture used for double contrast enemas.

Balloon-type catheters (Foley and similar) and rigid plastic enema nozzles should be avoided, unless specially asked for by the radiologist. Round-ended soft plastic catheters or rubber 'whistle-tip' catheters are both suitable. Use the largest size that can easily be introduced (8 or 10 for infants, 12 or 14 at 1 year old, 18 or 20 for 10 year olds).

Once the catheter has been introduced, infants and children under 3 years should have the buttocks taped together with sticky tape. Tubular elasticated bandage is useful to keep a baby's legs immobilized.

A nurse rather than a parent should accompany a baby, (or an older child who is to have a double-contrast enema.) She should stand at the head end of the table during screening and hold the baby's arms out of the x-ray field.

The screening technique is basically the same as for an adult, modified perhaps by the radiologist to suit the provisional diagnosis. Lateral film(s) of the rectum are taken for suspected Hirschsprung's disease, and a late after-evacuation film at some time between 6 and 24 h. Babies' barium enemas are given by 50-ml syringe.

Double-contrast enema

A small amount of barium is run into the colon under fluoroscopic control. The radiologist may decide to siphon back some of the barium, depending on how much has been used. The Higginson syringe is attached to the catheter and air introduced into the bowel. When enough air has been introduced the syringe is disconnected and the catheter end clamped with a forceps or clip.

Radiographs of the abdomen are taken with the overcouch tube. As the child may be in some discomfort, the series of films should be taken as quickly as possible. To facilitate this, everything should be got ready beforehand as follows:

(i)   a vertical cassette holder in place if available;

(ii)   if not, two 45° foam pads and sandbags;

(iii)   a grid and cassette of adequate size, probably 30 × 40 cm (15 × 12 in) Sellotaped together (or a grid-cassette);

(iv)   as many more cassettes the same size as will be needed for further views;

(v)   large rectangular foam pieces to raise the child off the table for horizontal beam projections;

(vi)   upright Bucky, if available, in place vertically at the right height.

Nurse can help to steady the child in the various positions if necessary.

The following are the usual projections (other views may be added or substituted):

(1)   *Supine AP view.*

The child is then turned on one side raised on foam pads. His abdomen should be touching the vertical grid-cassette.

(2)   *PA view, right or left lateral decubitus, with horizontal beam.*

The procedure is reversed: the child lies on the other side.

(3)   *AP view, left or right lateral decubitus, with horizontal beam.*

(4)   *Prone view of the lower abdomen* with 30° tilt to the feet to show the sigmoid colon.

(5)   *AP view erect.*

The films are speedily processed and checked by the radiologist. As soon as possible, the catheter is removed and the child put on a bedpan or sent to the toilet to relieve the discomfort of his distended bowel.

Exposure factors

A chart of exposure factors for infant, toddler and child having opaque swallow, meal or enema examination, should hang beside the control panel in the screening room so as to avoid the all too likely over- or underexposure due to guesswork. Relatively high kilovoltage is used (perhaps 70–85 kV). The exposure time must be as short as possible. The grid need not be used for infants.

It is particularly important to use a high kilovoltage in double contrast enemas so that the whole range of densities between the two extremes of contrast may be equally well visualized. A kilovoltage range of 90–100 kV, with perhaps 8–10 mAs, is suggested for a 10 year old.

CHAPTER 12

THE NEONATE

The term 'neonate' is applied to infants up to one month old. A 'premature baby' is one born before completion of a full-term pregnancy.

Radiography of these infants is a very responsible job which should not be entrusted to an inexperienced young radiographer except under supervision. It is extremely important that the films should be diagnostically adequate at first attempt; it is inexcusable to have to repeat them because of bad radiographic technique.

A general hospital with a maternity ward will usually have a special care baby unit to deal with medical cases. Those needing surgery are usually transferred to a children's hospital, as neonatal surgery is a highly specialized field. However, films to help in diagnosis or exclusion of a surgical emergency will be requested in the hospital where the baby is born.

Premature babies are always in an incubator and will be x-rayed with the mobile machine. Ill full-term babies are usually in an incubator, but may come to the department if it is easy to move the incubator there and be taken out briefly if the doctor in charge of the case permits.

INCUBATOR BABIES

General care

Warmth

All neonates lose heat very rapidly and can die from heat loss.

It is important to remember that the incubator provides warmth of 85°–90°, so do not open it for longer than is absolutely necessary. If the infant is to be taken out, the x-ray room must be warmed first and the infant wrapped in cotton wool or gamgee while he is out. Never put a cold cassette in contact with an infant's skin.

Sterility
Newborn infants have very little defence against infection. The incubator provides a germ-free atmosphere, so anything put into it, including your hands, must be scrupulously clean. In some special care units you will have to wear a gown and/or mask.

Handling
Handling should be kept to an absolute minimum. All sick neonates should be handled very gently. Premature babies with cardiac or respiratory abnormalities can arrest after being moved about too much. Infants with intestinal obstruction may be in acute distress and should be disturbed as little as possible.

Be most careful you *do not ever dislodge an intravenous drip*. It may well be an infant's life-line and may have been set up only after great difficulty. It will probably be in a scalp-vein.

Other tubes attached to baby or his surroundings may include:

(i)   naso-gastric tube (for feeding or aspiration of stomach contents);
(ii)   umbilical catheters (one in the vein, one in the artery, to obtain blood samples for analysis);
(iii)   rectal thermometer;
(iv)   electrocardiogram leads from various parts of body (attached to a heart-beat monitor);
(v)   endotracheal tube to respirator (used in acute respiratory distress);
(vi)   suction tube (for clearing upper airways);
(vii)   flex from apnoea mattress (an alarm is set off by this if the infant stops breathing);
(viii)   under-water seal (used for treatment of pneumothorax, see p. 35).

Some of these may leave the incubator through a slot beside the port-holes. Watch they do not get trapped or pulled when opening and closing the port-holes or the side flap. Do not jar the incubator or let the flap drop, or jerk it when moving it.

The bottle of the underwater seal will be at a lower level than the infant. It must never be raised higher (for instance, put on top of the incubator 'out of the way').

Tiny premature infants may be wrapped in tinfoil, or have head or body in a Perspex box. Do not remove anything used in the nursing care of the infant without prior permission from sister or staff nurse.

Hazards

Oxygen

Infants in respiratory distress may be on oxygen therapy. This should ideally be switched off for the duration of the x-ray exposure if a mobile machine is being used, but this may not always be possible.

Always ask permission first.

Radiation

It is the responsibility of the radiographer to make sure that any nurse holding an infant for x-ray examination is adequately protected with a lead apron and is not pregnant.

Artefacts

Apnoea mattress

The usual alarm mattress is like a mini air-bed. It is radio-opaque, showing up as a series of lines across the film. Put the cassette on top of it, or remove it.

Incubators

There is a *round hole* in the top of an incubator, sometimes with a metal mesh. Do not x-ray baby underneath this, as, even without the mesh, it will show up on a film as a round area of greater density. This can be very misleading over the lung fields or over the gut gas-pattern.

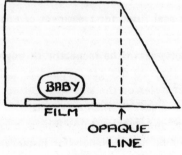

Fig. 71.

Some incubators have a *sloping side*. The angle made where this joins the top will appear on the film as an opaque line. Make sure baby and film are well clear of it (Fig. 71).

Tubes and leads
These are all more or less radio-opaque. Move them aside when possible.

PATHOLOGY

The chest
Respiratory distress syndrome (RDS)
Difficulty in breathing, occurring shortly after birth, is found mainly in premature infants. One of the commonest causes is *hyaline membrane disease*, in which the lining of the alveoli is abnormal. Other causes are: *congenital atelectasis* (failure of the lungs to expand fully) which can be followed by *lobar collapse*; and *pneumothorax*.

Congenital heart disease (CHD)
There are many forms of congenital heart disease caused by abnormalities of anatomy or physiology. Heart disease is quite common in the newborn.

There are two much rarer conditions which, though not arising in the lungs or heart, are demonstrable on a chest radiograph. Both are surgical emergencies.

Diaphragmatic hernia
An infant suffering from diaphragmatic hernia is born with part of the abdominal contents lying within the chest cavity, sometimes occupying the space normally taken up by an entire lung. Surgery to correct this is of the utmost urgency if the infant's life is to be saved.

Oesophageal atresia
Atresia means a lack of continuity of an anatomical tube. In the oesophagus there may be an associated fistula to the trachea. By far the commonest variant is shown in Fig. 72. As the upper oesophagus ends in a blind pouch, swallowed fluid will come back and some will be

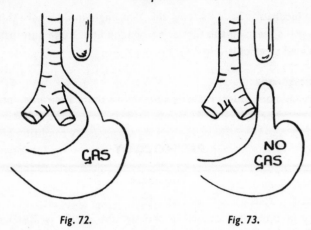

Fig. 72.   Fig. 73.

inhaled, causing breathing difficulty. The fistula between the trachea
and lower oesophagus will cause air to show in the stomach. A much
rarer form is illustrated in Fig. 73. It is important that the stomach is
included on the film to differentiate between these two conditions.

An opaque catheter is passed down the oesophagus as far as it will
go, before the chest radiograph is taken. It is not usually considered
necessary, or even wise, to use an opaque medium of any kind, because
of the danger of its being inhaled. AP and lateral views are taken of the
chest and upper abdomen.

The abdomen

Congenital abnormalities of the gastro-intestinal tract can occur at any
level from upper oesophagus to anus. They are not common; some are
very rare. But if they give rise to *obstruction*, early diagnosis and surgical
treatment are essential. Oesophageal atresia has been dealt with above.
Obstruction (of the intestine) beyond the stomach results in a request
for abdominal radiographs.

Duodenal atresia

Atresia of the duodenum is rare. A supine film demonstrates that there
are no gas shadows beyond the duodenum. An erect film gives the typical
'double bubble' appearance caused by air–fluid levels in the stomach
and in the duodenum.

Jejunal–ileal atresia
Also rare, it occurs anywhere along the length of the small gut. (Atresia of the colon is extremely rare.)

Malrotation and volvulus
'Malrotation' of the gut means that the small and large intestines have not taken up the correct anatomical position within the infant's abdomen. The bowel is thus predisposed to 'volvulus', the condition of being revolved or twisted on itself. Eventually, obstruction and strangulation result. Peristalsis triggers off the volvulus, so it does not appear until the infant is a few days old.

In the commonest variety of the abnormality, the caecum lies in the right hypochodrium and is attached to the lateral abdominal wall by peritoneal bands which may obstruct the duodenum, as well as possibly causing a volvulus in the small bowel.

Hirschsprung's disease
A congenital lack of ganglion cells in the intestine, which means that abnormal peristalsis produces intestinal obstruction. It may affect any part of the intestine, but most commonly rectum, or rectum and part of sigmoid. The obstruction usually presents soon after birth.

Imperforate anus
There are several anatomical variations. Basically this is a congenital lack of continuity between terminal gut and anal dimple.

Meconium ileus
Not strictly a congenital malformation, meconium ileus means a blockage of terminal ileum by thick meconium, due to an uncommon hereditary disease called cystic fibrosis.

Any of these conditions can result in complete or incomplete obstruction of gut shortly after birth.

RADIOGRAPHIC TECHNIQUE

Most requests for x-ray examination of neonates are for films of the chest and/or abdomen. Less often films are needed of limbs for birth injuries, and skull, spine or limbs for congenital malformations.

The chest

The mobile machine used for chest radiography of neonates must be capable of giving 0·02 s exposure time and at least 150 mA. Depending on baby's size, from 55 to 60 kV and 3 or 4 mAs, at a distance of 36–40 in, should give adequate AP films. These may be done supine or erect, according to the radiologist's preference. Premature and ill babies will be x-rayed supine in the incubator. In some hospitals two AP films are taken routinely, especially for the first examination. They are bound to be at different phases of inspiration, and one may confirm or exclude something seen on the other. Lateral projections are generally to be avoided, unless specially requested by the radiologist or paediatrician. They can be taken with the horizontal beam, baby supine, to avoid moving him. If catheters have been passed into the umbilical vein or artery (for blood studies) the chest films should include the upper abdomen to localize their position.

Some radiologists like the abdomen to be included routinely on the first films of a distressed neonate, as the cause of the respiratory difficulty may be abdominal rather than strictly thoracic. Take only one AP radiograph in this case, and show it to the radiologist or paediatrician before taking any further films.

In the ward

Get the x-ray machine in position, switch on, centre approximately. If there is a sandbag under baby's shoulders ask nurse to substitute a rolled paper towel or cottonwool. If he is lying on a slant, head either higher or lower than body, ask her to put him flat. Wipe the cassette with Savlon, cover it with a paper towel. Set the exposure factors, including distance. Put lead aprons on yourself and nurse. Do not open the incubator until you have everything ready.

AP supine

Work from the flap side of the incubator with nurse at the other side. Nurse puts her hands through the port-holes and lifts baby up. You open the flap and put a 13 × 18 cm (8 × 6 in) cassette crosswise on the alarm mattress. Shut the flap, open your port-holes to do final positioning. As nurse lowers baby on to the cassette be sure no catheter or electrocardiogram lead lies under him. Watch for all other hazards mentioned above, especially the hole in the incubator top. Right or left letter and name space on the cassette should be well clear of baby. The top edge of the cassette should be immediately under the infant's occiput, so it will need an extra fold of paper towel or a small cotton-wool 'cushion'. There is no need to extend an infant's arms or legs. Nurse holds the head and knees to keep the chest straight in the AP position. (Infants' heads, especially if they are premature, lie laterally; it is essential that nurse holds the head *absolutely* AP or the chest will not be.)

Close your port-holes when baby is positioned. Arms can be ignored, just wait until they are clear of the chest before exposing. Cone very carefully so that the x-ray field just includes the chest. Turn off the oxygen (if permitted). Run the anode: Watch the infant's respiration carefully; it may be very fast or erratic. You may have to wait a few minutes for baby to settle again after being disturbed. On inspiration a hollow dent appears just below the sternum: expose when you see this. Retrieve the cassette with equal care for all the points mentioned above.

If the film is to include the upper abdomen for location of umbilical catheters, use an 18 × 24 cm (10 × 8 in) cassette lengthwise, and extend the x-ray field to the level of the iliac crests.

Some incubators incorporate a film tray: the only handling of the infant that is necessary is to position and maintain him in the true AP position. Accurate centring of the film is more difficult in this case, so use an 18 × 24 cm (10 × 8 in) cassette rather than the 13 × 18 cm (8 × 6 in). Remember to remove the alarm mattress if it is the opaque type.

Recumbent lateral view

Technique is the same as for the supine AP view except that nurse lays the infant on his side on the film, and must hold the arms above the head as far as possible clear of the chest. This is not easy to do and will require careful positioning, as infants strongly resist having their arms (or legs) extended. If baby is very ill and this position too much of a strain on him, it is better to do the lateral projection with a horizontal beam and leave baby supine. It will be found less difficult to extend the arms when he is lying on his back.

Lateral view with horizontal beam
Centre the x-ray beam horizontally, between the port-holes. Put a
cassette in the incubator between the side of the incubator and the
edge of the tray that baby lies on. Nurse can hold his arms above his
head through the port-hole, standing at the head end (Fig. 74). There is
seldom need to hold his legs.

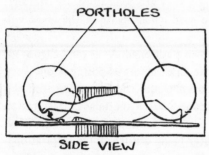
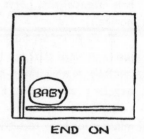

PORTHOLES

SIDE VIEW   END ON

Fig. 74.

In the x-ray department

It may be decided that baby is fit enough to be taken to the department
for x-ray examination either in, or out of, the incubator. If he is coming
in an incubator:

(i)   warm up the room beforehand;
(ii) keep him out of the incubator for minimum time;
(iii) do not uncover him until the last minute.

   The film may be taken supine AP, or erect PA or AP.

Supine AP and lateral views
Centre to a cassette covered with a folded paper towel on the x-ray
table: cone within its edges: set the exposure factors. Nurse holds baby
in position as previously described.

Erect AP view
It is very difficult to avoid a lordotic projection if baby's feet and buttocks
are on the same level. A baby chest-stand, as described in Chapter 2
(p. 25), is almost essential for the accurate radiography of these tiny
patients. They have an incredible ability to squirm out of a true AP
position. The pelvis must be firmly immobilized against the bottom edge

of the cassette with a Velcro strap. Nurse holds baby's elbows against his ears, and the head between, absolutely straight.

If you have no baby chest-stand, it is possible to utilize the screening-stand step at the end of the x-ray table. Sellotape the cassette against it, sit baby in front of it astride a 45° foam pad, with a sandbag against the outside of each thigh (Fig. 75). A 5° tilt down will compensate for any

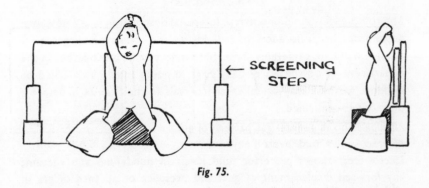

Fig. 75.

tendency to a lordotic position. Centre just under baby's chin, whether you tilt the tube or not. The lower edge of the x-ray field should come just below the nipple level. (A common mistake is to include half the abdomen on a chest film, see pp. 3 and 4.)

Erect PA view
Some radiologists insist on even neonatal chests being positioned PA, especially for heart size (opinions vary on this point).

In this case it is essential to have a special chest-stand. If something similar to the one described in Chapter 2 (p. 25) is available, it is useful to have various thicknesses of foam pads for the seat, to bring baby's chest up to the correct level.

To ensure the apices are on the film, the top cassette edge must be at the level of the baby's nose and mouth; extra care is needed to avoid damaging them. Nurse holds baby's arms and head as for the AP position, but must also extend at least two fingers of each hand round the back of baby's head or he will jerk it backwards. Cone to within the cassette edges. A Velcro strap across baby's lap will help to keep him straight and still (Fig. 14, p. 26).

Erect lateral view
Seat baby sideways to the cassette, Velcro strap across the thighs.
Nurse holds his left arm with her left hand, his right hand with her right.
(Reverse for left lateral.) Her wrist will then be behind his head to
support it (Fig. 15, p. 72).

The abdomen

The routine views to demonstrate intestinal obstruction in the newborn
depend on the preferences of radiologists and paediatric surgeons. A
minimum of two, preferably three, films is necessary; taken either in the
department or on the ward. Baby's age in hours should be marked on
all films, as these may be taken at intervals in the first 24 h before a
diagnosis is confirmed.

AP supine shows general gas pattern of gut.

AP erect shows fluid levels if any.

Lateral erect shows posterior fluid levels in duodenum and rectum;
any forward displacement of gut; and presence or absence of gas in
rectum.

Left lateral recumbent outlines the duodenum with gas.

Decubitus AP shows fluid levels in an infant too ill to be taken out of the
incubator for erect films.

Inverted lateral is usually taken only in cases of imperforate anus, but
some radiologists require inverted views in suspected Hirschsprung's
disease cases.

Lateral with horizontal beam (*patient supine*): in the extremely rare case
of a very ill infant with free air in the peritoneal cavity, this view will
demonstrate the condition adequately without disturbing him.

Remember you are dealing with a sick distressed infant who is
probably in considerable pain.

Treat him gently. Keep him warm.

The upper edge of the x-ray field is at the level of the nipples. The
lower edge is parallel with baby's bottom, an inch or so below (Fig. 76).
This ensures that the diaphragm and the whole of the rectum are on the
film. The use of a grid is optional.

With careful collimation it should be possible to avoid irradiating a
male infant's gonads. Lead protection is not really advisable as it can so
easily obscure important information.

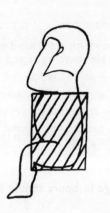 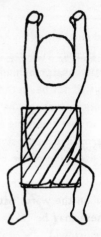

Fig. 76.

In the ward

AP view supine and *lateral view with horizontal beam (baby supine)*
The technique is much the same as for chests (p. 136–8) except that:

(i)   it is not so important to hold the head absolutely straight;

(ii)   0·04 s is the maximum exposure time;

(iii)   infants with abdominal pain draw their knees up, so it would be even more than usually difficult to straighten the legs. Do not try: nurse can hold the ankles. Again there is no need to raise the arms, just watch that they are out of the way before exposing.

Recumbent lateral view
It is not necessary to get the arms above the head as for a chest film (Fig. 77). Be sure the infant is exactly lateral, not oblique.

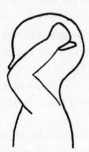 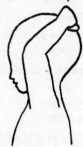

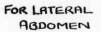

FOR LATERAL   FOR LATERAL
ABDOMEN   Fig. 77.   CHEST

Erect AP view

With care and the help of an experienced nurse, it is possible to sit an infant on the opened side-flap of his incubator, with a film Sellotaped upright to the incubator behind him. He must be raised on something, or the rectum will not be on the film. A folded nappy will do, or a small polystyrene block, such as the Conray pack) The cassette should be upside down, so that the name space is at the bottom of the film. Nurse holds baby's arms and head, standing beside, not behind him. The legs are abducted, each side of the block (Fig. 78).

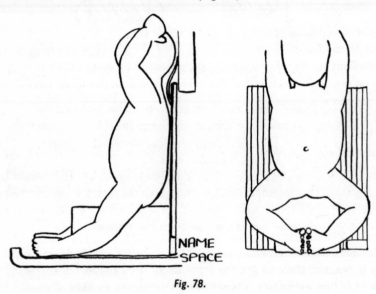

Fig. 78.

Erect lateral view

This is taken in the same way. Leave the block in the same position, sit baby sideways on it, not astride, so his pelvis and abdomen are in the true lateral position to the film (Fig. 79).

Lateral with horizontal beam (baby supine) and *lateral decubitus (AP view) with horizontal beam*

These further views may be taken instead of the erect views, or to give additional information. The cassette is vertical between the tray and the incubator side. Raise baby by placing a folded nappy under him (see 'lateral chest with horizontal beam', p. 138).

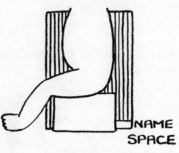

Fig. 79.

In the x-ray department
Erect AP and lateral views
These films can be taken in the baby chest-stand by using a thicker foam
pad on the seat to ensure the rectum is included on the films. Baby sits
astride the seat. The Velcro strap goes round it and his legs, just below
the knees.

Lacking a baby chest-stand, use the screening stand step: Sellotape
a cassette against it vertically. Sit baby in front of it, astride a 45° foam
pad with sandbags against the outside of each leg, as described before
for erect chest radiography (see p. 139). Be careful of the leg and foot
nearest the cassette when positioning for the lateral view.

Inverted lateral view
This view should not be taken by dangling an infant upside down by the
legs in front of the chest-stand: his head must be supported correctly.
The 'dangling' technique is more likely to produce an oblique view.

The infant must be at least 18 h old, preferably 24 h. He should be
held upside down on nurse's lap for 10–15 min before the film is taken
(Fig. 80).

A chair or stool is placed in front of the (adult) chest stand, with a
foam ring or block on the seat for baby's head to rest on. Nurse, in
lead–rubber coat, stands at the side and holds him by the knees, not the
ankles.

It is essential that baby's pelvis is exactly at right angles to the film
for a true lateral projection. Measurements are made on this radiograph,
so positioning must be extremely accurate. It may be considered easier
to achieve this if the infant's legs are at right angles to the body. Either

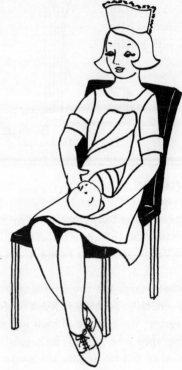

Fig. 80.

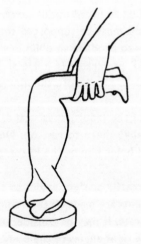 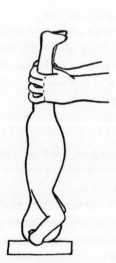

Fig. 81.

method of holding can be utilized, provided an exact true lateral view is produced (Fig. 81). Sometimes it is requested that the anal dimple is localized on the film with a metal marker.

AP supine and Recumbent lateral views are taken as for chest, see p. 141.

Congenital abnormalities

Arrange with the ward to let you have the infant just after a feed. Sleep is the best of all methods of immobilization.

Skull or spine

Take AP and lateral views, preferably with a grid. If the abnormality includes a soft tissue swelling, choose exposure factors to demonstrate it as well as bony defects. (See also 'spina bifida' p. 96.)

Limbs

Usually only one view of both arms or both legs is required, either AP or lateral, whichever shows the abnormalities most clearly.

CHAPTER 13

SPECIAL INVESTIGATIONS

SKELETAL SURVEY FOR NON-ACCIDENTAL INJURY

In view of the horrifying number of 'battered baby' cases that have come to light in recent years, it is now fairly widely accepted that any baby under a year old with a fractured limb or skull should have a full skeletal survey to discover if there are other recent or healed fractures.

It is possible to fit a small baby all on one 35 × 43 cm (17 × 14 in) cassette; it is difficult, but not impossible, to ensure all four limbs and trunk are in a true AP position at the same time; up to about 6–8 weeks the same exposure factors will show ribs, spine and limb bones.

However, it is easier to achieve good positioning and immobilization if you x-ray the baby in two halves.

Thorax and upper limbs

Lay baby on a 24 × 30 cm (12 × 10 in) cassette with a small piece of foam under the head and back where the cassette edges come (Fig. 82). Immobilize the baby's lower half with the compression band. The hands and wrists are held AP: Sellotape across the wrists may be helpful. The head must be kept in the AP position. If it turns to either side the mandible will be superimposed on the clavicle. The name-space must not obscure the wrist or elbow. All epiphyses must be clearly shown: the ends of long bones are commonly injured.

Pelvis and lower limbs

Remove nappy. Place baby prone on a 24 × 30 cm (12 × 10 in) cassette as in Fig. 83. Immobilize with the compression band across his bottom (not too tightly). The toes of each foot are held so that the whole length of each leg from ankle to hip is PA.

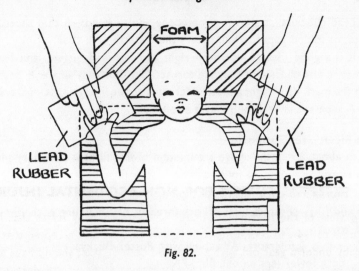

Fig. 82.

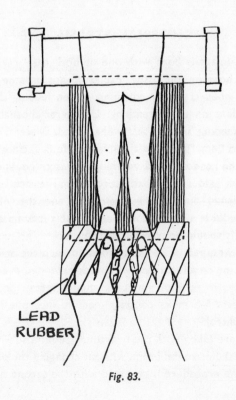

Fig. 83.

Lead cut-outs, as shown, protect the adult's hands. A thin sheet of foam, or folded paper towel, covers the cassette each time.

It is a good idea to use both right and left lead letters, and have someone else check that they are correct. The films may appear in court, and the marking of right and left sides must not be in any doubt whatever.

A separate lateral skull film is also taken.

Children over 2 months

From about 2 months of age a minimum of five films is necessary plus the lateral skull film, as follows:

(i)   thorax and upper arms, AP supine;

(ii) and (iii)   separate films of each forearm AP, including both elbows and wrists;

(iv)   pelvis and femora, AP supine with Potter–Bucky;

(v)   both lower legs on one film, PA.

CHOANAL ATRESIA

Very rarely an infant is born with one or both nasal cavities blocked posteriorly by bone or soft tissue. Babies do not breathe through the mouth except when crying or coughing. When feeding they are completely dependent on nose-breathing. Unilateral choanal atresia may result in slow feeding, or may pass undiagnosed. Bilateral atresia, however, is a surgical emergency, as the infant's life is endangered.

The diagnosis is confirmed radiologically by the injection of an opaque medium under fluoroscopic control. The nose needs to be thoroughly cleaned out first, in the ward, and the infant sedated. Ultrafluid Lipiodol is a suitable medium for this examination, because it flows easily. It should be warmed before use.

The infant, wrapped in a small blanket to keep the arms out of the way, is laid supine on a foam pad, with neck extended over the edge so that the head is in position for a sub-mento-vertex projection. The radiologist injects 3–5 ml of contrast medium into one nostril under fluoroscopic control.

Two views are taken with the overcouch tube: a sub-mento-vertex and a lateral with horizontal beam, without changing the position of the baby's head. The procedure is repeated with the second nostril.

ORTHODONTICS

The orthodontist is concerned with the correction of dental malocclusion, a word which means literally 'bad closing'. An abnormal bite (e.g. protruding upper front teeth) occurs if the upper and lower jaws do not match in size. Crowding of the teeth results if the jaw is too small to accommodate them.

Orthodontic treatment may involve the extraction of certain teeth to allow more space for the remainder, and/or the wearing of an appliance (usually intra-oral) designed to adapt the dental arches gradually over a period of months. The orthodontist will also recommend surgical treatment for any permanent teeth which are erupting in the wrong place or at the wrong angle, and the removal of supernumary teeth.

Children are usually referred about 7 or 8 years of age, when the dental abnormalities first become obvious. X-ray examination of both jaws is required at this first visit to demonstrate the presence and position of all unerupted teeth and any pathological condition.

A single panoramic view of both jaws on one film is provided by a specially-designed tomographic machine such as the Orthopantomograph, if one is available.

(The technique for using this machine is not described, as the best way to learn how to use it is by demonstration.)

The same information can be provided for the orthodontist by three radiographs:

(1)   standard occlusal film to show the upper incisors and canines;
(2) and (3)   lateral oblique jaw views (sometimes called 'bimolar' views). Both sides are x-rayed always. The technique is the same as for the standard view of the body (not the ramus) of the mandible, with slight modifications:

(i)   the neck and chin are extended to remove the mandible as far as possible from superimposition by the cervical spine;

(ii)   the head is rotated forwards, from the standard position, until the nose and chin touch the cassette (13 × 18 cm (8 × 6 in) used transversely) (Fig. 84). The jaws are closed.

The simplest way of standardizing these projections is by using a 35° angle board in the chest stand. The films can then be taken erect. If no

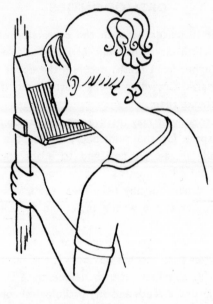

Fig. 84.

angle board is available, it may be possible to get one made, fixed at an angle of 35°, with a ledge to support the cassette. This eliminates the necessity to tilt the tube. Centring is over the mastoid process remote from the film. The x-ray field is limited to within the edges of the cassette A long sinus cone may be used to reduce scattered radiation.

The radiographs should show the whole of the lower *and upper* teeth as far as the canines, free from superimposition by the other side.

PA and lateral skull views

These views may also be required to locate any abnormally positioned teeth (e.g. buried maxillary canines) and to show the precise relationship of the teeth to the jaws and other structures in the skull.

The orthodontist does not really mean 'skull' as a radiographer understands the word. The *base* of the skull, from frontal sinus to occipital protuberance, should be shown on the lateral view, for measurement points. The *vault* of the skull is not usually required. Similarly, the PA 'skull' film is really a PA view of mandible and maxillae: again the vault of the skull is not needed.

The craniostat (cephalostat) is used for these views, if available. It consists of a framework to hold the patient's head in standard PA and lateral positions by means of earplugs and a nasal or forehead rest. There is an attachment to hold a cassette. The complete craniostat incorporates an immovable x-ray tube at 6-ft focal-film distance, centred permanently to the cassette holder so that the opaque earplugs are always super-imposed in the lateral view.

There is also an aluminium wedge filter to enable a soft tissue profile of the face to be visualized in the lateral view.

Your x-ray department may have a complete cephalostat, or one without a fixed x-ray tube, or you may be asked to provide these views as accurately as possible without any specialized equipment.

Lateral view

An 18 × 24 cm (10 × 8 in) cassette and grid are put in the chest-stand, at the correct height for the seated patient. The tube is centred to the cassette from 6-ft distance. The head is positioned as accurately as possible in a true lateral position. The central ray should pass through the temporo-mandibular joints. The chin is extended slightly: on the resultant radiograph the Frankfurt line should appear parallel to the bottom edge of the film. A soft tissue profile of the face can be shown on this film, if it is required, by the following methods:

(i) using a strip of lead foil (the thickness depends on the kilovoltage used), stuck to the edge of the cassette behind the child's profile;

(ii) off-setting the grid slightly towards the back of the child's head, so that the profile comes just beyond the edge of the grid and the coincident light beam diaphragm.

In using either of these methods, care must be taken not to include the top central incisors in the soft tissue profile. This requires very accurate adjustment if, as often happens, these teeth protrude.

(iii) It is possible by trial and error to arrive at exposure factors which, without a grid, will demonstrate both facial skeleton and soft tissue profile.

PA view

Positioning and centring are the same as for a standard PA view of the mandible, again at 6-ft focal-film distance. A sufficiently high kilovoltage is chosen to demonstrate adequately the upper central incisors through the superimposed cervical spine.

Earrings, neckchains, etc., should, of course, be removed in all skull radiography. The patient should also be asked if he is wearing an intra-oral appliance, as this should also be removed before x-ray examination.

AIR VENTRICULOGRAPHY OF INFANTS

In the maternity unit of a general hospital, the problem occasionally arises of a newborn baby with a rapidly enlarging head. The usual cause of this condition is *hydrocephalus*. Normally, cerebro-spinal fluid is produced in the brain, circulates, and is reabsorbed continuously. The rates of production and reabsorption are exactly matched. If the flow or absorption is obstructed, the cerebro-spinal fluid accumulates, the ventricles become dilated and the skull expands.

The diagnosis of enlarged ventricles is confirmed by air ventriculo-graphy. The cause of the obstruction may be revealed only by further more specialized techniques. All the investigations, therefore, should be done at a specialized unit, where both diagnosis and treatment can be undertaken.

However, there are occasions when the x-ray department of the hospital where the infant is born may be requested to perform an air ventriculogram.

Air (or oxygen) is introduced into a lateral ventricle by direct puncture through the anterior fontanelle. A strictly aseptic technique is used. General anaesthesia is not necessary but the infant should be well sedated.

Six films are usually taken, a seventh if it is considered essential to attempt demonstration of the third and fourth ventricles. The centring is higher than for conventional skull films, as it is only the brain which is of interest: the facial bones and jaw are not.

AP, Townes and lateral with horizontal beam views
These views are taken with the infant supine. The films must all be checked by the radiologist before proceeding further.

If they are satisfactory, the infant is turned prone. Separate foam pads support the trunk and forehead, leaving a space between so that the infant can breathe.

PA, reverse Towne's and lateral with horizontal beam views are then taken, and shown to the radiologist.

'Hanging head' lateral view
The third and fourth ventricles may be visualized by laying the infant supine, with the body raised on foam pads, and the neck extended so that the head is in position for a submento-vertex projection. Fold the ears forward and tape with Sellotape. A *lateral* view with horizontal beam is then taken, centred just behind the folded ear.

In moving the infant from one position to another, the head must not be jerked or jolted. Manoeuvres of the head, to attempt to fill unvisualized parts of the ventricular system with air, must not be carried out by anyone who does not have precise knowledge of exactly what he or she is doing.

HYDROCEPHALUS WITH SHUNT

Hydrocephalus is treated with a shunt system which drains excess cerebro-spinal fluid from the ventricles of the brain into the right atrium of the heart (or less often, into the peritoneal cavity). The operation to insert the system is performed as soon as the diagnosis of hydrocephalus is confirmed, often as early as three weeks of age.

The Holter shunt

The Holter shunt is the system most widely used in this country (Fig. 85). It consists of two radio-opaque catheters with a valve between. The valve is metal, with a plastic centre. To the top metal end is attached the proximal catheter which then passes through a burr-hole into the right lateral ventricle of the brain. To the bottom end is attached the distal catheter which passes subcutaneously to the internal jugular vein into which it is inserted, thus reaching the heart. If this catheter is lengthened or changed at any time, it is reconnected by a small metal connector at the point of insertion into the jugular vein.

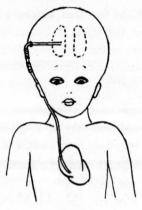

Fig. 85.

Any of these connections can come adrift causing the system to cease functioning, with consequent raised intra-cranial pressure; or, with the child's growth, the distal catheter may have become too short and lie in the superior vena cava, with the same result.

The child will usually be attending at intervals the specialized hospital at which the valve was originally inserted. However, this may be too far away if an emergency situation arises through failure of the shunt and the child may well arrive at the nearest emergency centre.

The x-ray request form will probably ask for skull and chest films. This does *not* mean the usual three skull views for accident cases, nor 6-ft erect films for lungfields. What is needed is a radiographic demonstration of the whole length of the shunt system. In particular, that part of each catheter immediately adjacent to the valve (and any connector) must be clearly seen.

Skull

AP (not PA) view

Include as much of the neck as possible. The vertical first part of the catheter, where it joins the valve, may be obscured by dense bone. Or it may be completely 'blacked out' where it overlies soft tissue. Additional oblique views will be necessary, coned to the area of the valve.

(1) A tangential projection, rotating the head (from the AP position)

away from the valve will bring it into profile. Reduce the kilovoltage. The connection of catheter and lower end of valve should be seen. Sometimes the upper end can be seen, but if not take the following view also.
(2)   To show the connection of catheter and upper end of valve rotate the head from the AP position *towards* the valve. The amount of rotation is judged from the AP film. The object is to project the valve to overlie the parietal bone.

Lateral view
The cassette should be used lengthwise, not transversely, in the Bucky tray, so as to include the neck.

It is important to demonstrate the junctions of catheters and valve in two projections. Either end may be disconnected.

Chest
It is not strictly the chest which is to be x-rayed, but the heart and as much of the distal catheter as can be included. There should be overlap between the AP skull and AP chest radiographs, so as to be sure of showing a possible metal connector in the neck area, again a likely disconnection site.

AP and lateral views
These are taken with the patient lying on the x-ray table, using a focal-film distance of 48 in (125 cm) or more. The exposure time needs to be very short: 0·02 or 0·03 s. Heart beat can blur the end of the catheter. The kilovoltage should be high enough to penetrate the heart shadow adequately, but the lungfields should not be obliterated.

Centring is over the heart, to give an accurate assessment of the exact position of the catheter end, in case it is no longer within the heart. Lead–rubber protection is used below the level of the heart.

The Pudenz shunt
A less frequently used system, the Pudenz shunt, is not radio-opaque except for the metal marker at the further tip of each catheter. Therefore, all that can be localized on a film is the position of the end of each catheter, and radiography is not much help in the case of malfunction of the system.

INDEX